Health

A Common "Sensible"
Approach

Martin S. Gildea, DC

Certified Functional Medicine Practitioner

❖

Create Space Publishing

Health:
A Common
"Sensible" Approach

Copyright 2014 Martin Gildea
All Rights Reserved

MEDICAL DISCLAIMER: The following information is intended for general information purposes only. Individuals should always consult their health care provider before administering any suggestions made in this book. The fact that an organization or website is referred to in this work as a citation and/or a potential source for further information does not mean that the Author endorses the information the organization or website may provide or recommendations in may make. Further, readers should be aware that internet websites listed in this work may have changed or disappeared between when this work was written and when it was read.

ISBN: 9781494232702

Library of Congress Control Number: 2014901224

INTENDED USE STATEMENT

All of the material written in this book is intended for informational purposes only and is not to be used in any way to diagnose, treat, cure or prevent any disease. The book attempts to emphasize nutritionally significant information. Healthy choice suggestions are made to support   health maintenance.

DISCLAIMER AND NOTICES

The contents of this book are not intended to be a substitute for personalized medical advice. The reader should seek a qualified health care provider. The suggestions in this book are based on alternative methods of nutrition and are not necessarily mainstream. The reader has the sole responsibility of choosing how they wish to implement any of the information contained therein and the discretion to see if any of the nutritional suggestions made are appropriate for them. The author of this information cannot be held responsible for interpretation of this information or for any unintentional misleading or omissions of the information.

The contents of this book should not be misinterpreted as a claim or representation in which any product mentioned or procedure constitutes a cure- palliative or ameliorative. All of the procedures discussed therein along with any nutritional protocols should be considered as alternative or adjunctive to other accepted conventional procedures deemed necessary by the attending licensed physician.

There are no nutritional compounds in this book meant to replace established, medical conventional approaches-especially in serious life threatening diseases or emergencies. None of the contents of this book have been evaluated by the Food and Drug Administration and the nutritional information contained therein is not meant to diagnose, treat, cure, or prevent disease.

<u>DEDICATION</u>

First, most importantly, I would like to dedicate this book to my family: my parents for giving me the love of books and education with an insatiable thirst for learning, my wife, Becky, for enduring my long hours on the computer studying which enabled me to write this book and may have taken me away from other activities, and to my two daughters, Alexis and Celina, who are both in college and grew up enduring my constant health advice and dietary restrictions.

Second, I wanted to dedicate this book to Dr. Mike Johnson from the Johnson group, as well as all of the chiropractors who comprise his message board. Dr. Johnson inspired me to write this book and much of the information contained therein was obtained from him and the many of the members of his board. They possess some the sharpest minds in all of chiropractic, bar none!

Third, I would like to dedicate this book to all of those chiropractors, who have been, and continue to be frustrated because we only see such a small percentage of the public due to medical misinformation. I wanted to give all chiropractors a voice here.

Contents

INTRODUCTION

So here we are in the winter of 2013 on a breezy, but uncharacteristically nice day for January 18th taking our dog Rufus for a walk at the Heritage War Museum Grounds in Carlisle, PA. Shortly after beginning the walk today we ran into a family on bicycles. The parents of this family looked younger than we were, and their kids looked to be in the 9-12 year range. When I first noticed them, they were coming to an abrupt halt on their bikes, stopping right in the middle of the path we were just about to take. The mother and the two kids were very out of breath. Keep in mind that we were only a few minutes from the parking lot, where they just unloaded their bikes. Becky and I both joked about how these kids could be tired so quickly, and while riding a bike to boot. Then upon closer inspection, I realized that the whole family was overweight and would be considered obese by today's standards. I immediately imagined seeing the kids play video games while their parents watched TV after eating a fast food meal or some microwavable pre-packaged concoction.

This also reminded me of a discussion I had a few days ago about why so many people in this country in such poor health. We all hear often about childhood obesity and how Michelle Obama wants to "nip it in the bud" so to speak and is trying to set an example with her vegetable garden and with the foods eaten in the White House. The statistics are shocking to hear: if people do not change their lifestyles including diet and exercise, this will be the first time in history when the current generation's parents will outlive their offspring.

As a practicing holistic chiropractor, I constantly deal with a confused public who are simply given the wrong nutritional information. Time and time again, I hear people cite the flawed food pyramid and that you should have six to seven servings of whole (wheat) grains per day and four to six servings of dairy including cow's milk. I am aware that people need to be educated enough to make decisions for themselves. As Dr. Mike Johnson, the leader of the Johnson Group said, "don't drink the Kool-Aid," a reference to Jonestown South Africa when the cult followers were instructed by leader Jim Jones to drink the Kool-Aid laced with poison. This is an extremely important issue because the food industry is a multi-billion dollar conglomerate. Some of the confusing food claims on the labels, and the deceptive advertising exhaust the patience of many who say "the hell with all of it" continue to eat processed foods that taste the best, are the cheapest, and the most profitable for them to make. Consequently, over 50% of the people in this country suffer from some type of chronic illness or condition, and over one third of this country is considered obese with a total body fat of 30% or over.

Thus I have decided to debunk some of these nutritional falsehoods. I will to tell you what I do in my life and what I believe anyone could do to have a better life. I will explain what you need to do in hopes of avoiding future chronic diseases and reach some sensible health goals.

Although I will try to keep this simple, I will often repeat the same information, some it technical but necessary in a different context. Hopefully, this will allow you to better understand how your body works and the adverse effects of putting all of the processed junk into it. There are a lot of different specialists in the medical field from internists and gastroenterologists to rheumatologists etc., keep in mind, however, that all of these specialists compartmentalize the human body into different areas to be treated separately. Yet, when talking about human physiology, all body systems are interrelated. It is impossible to treat or affect one area of the human body without affecting other areas. The human body is an incredible machine and one must, therefore, take a holistic (whole body) approach to truly understand and treat it successfully.

So eat (or better yet drink) your dark leafy green vegetables, put on your thinking cap, curl up on a chair and start reading. Remember, we are all looking for a magic bullet when it comes to health but people NEED to know there is no such thing. So let us begin...

<u>CHAPTER ONE</u>

Growing Up In a Health Conscious Environment

I would first like to tell you a little about my childhood and how I grew up and became a holistic chiropractor. I grew up in Bloomsburg, PA, which is a small town about 90 minutes north east of Harrisburg, PA, the state capital. My parents are both well educated. My mother has a master's degree in English and was a substitute high school teacher and my father was a political science professor at Bloomsburg University. I would consider my childhood normal as childhood's go. My dad would work during the day and read a lot when he came home. My mother did not teach when we were little and was a traditional housewife raising my brother, sister and me.

My parents were always health minded I would say. My dad did his share of beer drinking as he grew up in the coal region in Mount Carmel, PA - it was expected of him. I remember a recent conversation with my mother in which she told me about how important the bars were in the social life of those living in that area at the time. She said it was all about how much liquor, particularly beer, one could hold. The stories these guys today reminisce about somehow always include beer-drinking capacity. In fact my mother let me know again just the other day how my late uncle could drink a case of beer one day and then then next day go to work without a hangover.

My father walked to work every day up three huge hills. A half a mile or so of his walk was straight up. I am not kidding about the steepness of these hills. During one of my driver's lessons, I remember the instructor had me stop the car on the middle of one of the hills and put the emergency brake on. He then told me to release the brake and climb the hill. I will never forget how far and fast the car coasted backwards before going forward. This car was an automatic too. I laid some serious rubber! So my dad really was getting a cardio workout for many years. He walked up there for thirty plus years while teaching and continues to do so today at the age of 80. He basically ate what my mother would cook as most husbands did, and still do, if they cook that is?

My mother was a stay at home mom, as I said, who did not have a driver's license. She would trek a lot of miles on those legs over the years. She would also go up the hills and use the college gym to exercise. When we were little she would push us in the stroller and when we were old enough we would all walk. Ever since my siblings and I moved out of the house after college, she has probably walked and exercised at least five days per week.

Thus my parents were not couch potatoes. This reminds me of a funny story. I just recently went to my 30th high school reunion and could not believe how many of my classmates came up to me to ask about my mom and dad's health. They told of how they see my parents walking through and around town just about every day. I vividly remember how impressed they were when they were telling me this. Mom and dad are both in great shape and remain very trim to this day. To me it is only logical that you have to keep moving or the body wants to stiffen and then moving will be impossible.

My brother, sister, and I rode our bikes everywhere also when we were kids. And we played with the neighborhood kids and would not go home until my mom would whistle for us at 6pm each night. Thus the issue of exercise was not an issue back when I grew up in the seventies. There were no video games and very few people had cable TV. As you know this is not the case today.

When I look back on my childhood in terms of what my family ate, I think my mother did a great job. She is 100% Italian and always thought of food as the best medicine. However, the thing I appreciate the most about those days is the fact that my mom intuitively knew about the balance when preparing meals. We always had a protein and lots of vegetables with each meal unlike the simple carbohydrate sugary microwavable concoctions people call dinner today. We also were not milk drinkers like some of my friends who went through gallons per week. Desert was also rare in our diet. We did not get ice cream or get to drink soda very often. My mother was a little vain as she confessed to me many times. Since my father was a professor, which always involved many young beautiful girls, my mother joked she did not want to let herself get out of shape. She said the thought of the young college girls was good motivation to remain fit. After all, health and fitness all comes down to some type of motivation. People need to find what motivates them and tap into it.

Ever since I can remember my mom and dad always have and continue to read the New York Times. The health section would often give great advice and she would follow it. As a matter of fact even today I still get articles from my mom in the mail about a certain gene being discovered or concerning some controversial nutrition topic. So when it came to antibiotics and other over the counter, as well as prescription drugs, we only used them sparingly as we were hardly ever sick anyway. The stage was being set for me to go the "alternative "route.

Then there was the day that really changed my life and ultimately led me down the path of being a holistic practitioner. I was probably thirteen or so and my dad went on a shopping trip with the other professor husbands to get the family Christmas presents. To make a long story short, he brought me back a book called "The Education of a Bodybuilder" by Arnold Schwarzenegger. I saw the picture of his bicep on the cover and I was so amazed. I wanted to be powerful like this guy. Thus I started to workout sporadically and then when I was fifteen years old, I decided to get more serious. Since that time I have continued to work out for the past thirty-three years. I even entered a few natural bodybuilding contests and actually judged a couple during this time.

What the bodybuilding did for me was give me discipline. This discipline parlayed into the rest of my life. I still remember, as if it were yesterday, the day I hurt my upper back during the summer after my freshman year in college. I was at my buddy Dave's Stone Castle Gym doing front squats; all of a sudden I pulled a muscle in upper back and could not get a breath without a sharp stabbing pain in my side. I lay around on the couch that evening and most of the next day barely able to move; it was time to go to the emergency room. Let me say that nobody in our family was a pansy. The intern, who had been on staff at the hospital, never even touched me and almost acted as if I were an annoyance. He simply looked at me and told me to "put heat on it and take some Advil". In other words, going to the emergency room that day was just a waste of time. Soon I was back on the couch for three more days. Finally, I remembered someone at the gym telling me to try a chiropractor. I never heard of chiropractic before and had no idea what it even was. As I said, we hardly ever went to the doctors when I was growing up. It just so happened that a guy who graduated high school a couple of years ahead of me was the son of a chiropractor across the street from us. I really did not know him, but I was desperate to try anything.

The chiropractor looked a little older than my dad and was a very soft spoken man who sat me down and asked me some questions. He seemed to really listen and to care about what I had to say. He then felt around my back and told me to relax. What impressed me, is that he just squeezed a few areas on my ribcage; it only took a minute. I got up and walked out of there feeling 50% better. I was so amazed at the results that I questioned a chiropractor I met at my gym. Since

I worked out with the owner, I had ample chances to talk to this chiropractor, also was a gym member. He went to a school called Sherman in Spartanburg, South Carolina. I wanted to know what it entailed to become a chiropractor. When I learned that they were a drug free profession, it really clicked with me, as I grew up that way anyway. I was always oriented to a natural lifestyle that bodybuilding training had given me; no junk food, little alcohol, low processed sugar, and a lot of healthy fats, proteins, and veggies. Throw in the "religiously working out" component and I figured, hey, I already live the lifestyle so it should not be too hard? My father, the voice of reason, did tell me that the American Medical Association was very skeptical and biased against chiropractors. Of course at the time I did not understand this, but as time went on, boy did I ever come to realize what he meant by that statement.

CHAPTER TWO

My Career Epiphany

Before my career choice epiphany, I was going to be a business major. In retrospect that would have been a huge mistake. I am glad it all turned out the way that it did; I am NOT a businessman. After many discussions with other prospective chiropractic students I decided to apply to Palmer College in Davenport, Iowa, for the class of 1986. It was also during this time I met my future roommate, Neil Engelman, at Bloomsburg State College. It was amazing that two kids from the same small college were going to travel 850 miles away to be chiropractors and at the same time no doubt. After our undergraduate study was completed, Neil and I were off to Davenport Iowa in June of 1986.

During Chiropractic school, I stayed true to my bodybuilding training and never missed a workout. I studied hard and graduated with a B.S. in Biology along with the Doctorate of Chiropractic degree. It was during my second year that I met my wife Becky who was working as a waitress. Of course being the shy guy that I was, my additional roommates-from New York went up to Becky and sprung the news to her about my affection. You know how subtle and soft-spoken the New York guys can be. They used to call me Maaaaaaaty. Evidently there are no "r" letters pronounced in many of certain New Yorkers' vocabulary.

I used to cook food from scratch in Davenport while most of the other guys made pre-packaged noodles or just ate out at restaurants every day. I was spoiled from the bodybuilding lifestyle so, since there was no mom at college, I had to cook. I remember one of the New York students living across the hall in our apartment building, as there were no dorms at Palmer. He sat down to my home cooked Italian meal of spaghetti and meatballs; I actually made the sauce and meatballs from scratch. Of course the New Yorkers, all Italians, loved my cooking. One of them said, "Maaaaty you are going to make a good wife someday." I do miss those days of lower stress and a lot of fun; I loved school and hated for it to end, but knew I had to start paying the loans back.

During my life as a chiropractic student, I noticed a lot of soon to be doctors did not "walk the talk," so to speak. They did not eat right or exercise and really were poor examples of health. Their excuse was there was not enough time in a day to exercise and eat right, the same excuses the overweight general public still uses. I thought this odd but figured, since I was a bodybuilder, I was more serious about proper food and exercise than the average person. I would see these guys coming back late every night from the bars, usually pretty intoxicated. Exercise and preparing the proper foods would have interfered with their excessive party time. On the other hand, I would only go to a bar or parties on weekends if I went at all. During this time the discipline to not get caught up in all of the frivolous partying was reinforced.

Looking back, I realized the metabolic or nutritional aspect of health was not emphasized in my chiropractic education. Most of my metabolic/nutritious knowledge would come from continuous postgraduate course study and from real life experience with my own training.

For those of you who never heard of chiropractic or who know very little about what it is, I will briefly describe the art and science of it. Chiropractic was founded on the principles of "subluxation" in which there is a spinal bone out of place causing a problem with the nerve which courses along those particular vertebrae; this will affect the organ or tissue that this impinged nerve supplies. There are 24 spinal bones, and the spinal cord runs down through the center of each with a left and a right branch emanating out between each vertebra, one to the left and one to the right. This is much like a tree with left and right branches from top to bottom. The nerves in the neck supply areas from the neck and head but also down the upper extremities. The middle back nerves travel to organs and structures in the torso; the nerves in the lower back travel to the pelvic structures and to the lower extremities. The first chiropractic "adjustment," in which the chiropractor used his hands and the spinous process of the vertebrae as a lever to apply a high velocity force, was performed in 1895 by Dr. BJ Palmer. This patient was a deaf janitor who had his hearing restored after having vertebrae in his spine "racked". The chiropractic curriculum consists of thousands of hours of study, actually more hours than a medical doctor's degree, but does not include any residency or pharmaceutical training.

Today chiropractic has come a long way. There still are the "straight" chiropractors who only use their hands to adjust the spine. However, there are also the "mixer" chiropractors, who also use physical therapy techniques along with nutrition to treat patients. Chiropractic literally means "hand practice" and is not intended to treat any particular condition; it is supposed to balance the body systems by removing any interference, and thus restoring the normal nerve flow to the target tissue or organ. These imbalances are caused by physical, chemical, or emotional stressors. Theoretically, if the chiropractor can remove any imbalances, the human body can self-regulate and is in a state of homeostasis (balance). However somewhere along the way most modern day mixer chiropractors have been relegated to treating only back and neck pain probably because the vehicle of treatment is the spine, residing at the back and neck. More on this topic later in the treatment recommendation section of this book.

During my first quarter in school, I noticed one morning my left big toe was numb. This was no surprise, since I was training daily in gym with heavy weights. When I visited the assigned clinic doctor, he said "that is the left L4 nerve root in your lower back." The L4 nerve root innervates or gives energy to the big toe for both feeling and sensation or sensory input and for muscle function and motor input. The clinician put me on my side and did some "chiropractic maneuver" with an ensuing pop from the left lower back. I stood up and there was some immediate sensation returning to my left big toe. Within minutes it was totally normal; I was amazed.

When I began my clinical part of chiropractic school I was very nervous to say the least. Even today, I am always asked what it was like when I was learning "how to do this". My reply has always been the same: I tended, like my classmates, to not to use enough force during the procedure because of the apprehension a student usually feels. I remember one clinic doctor who used to tell me, "You are a strong weightlifter, why are you having so much trouble with this?" My buddies and I were simply too timid at first but once we got the confidence, we all became very good at adjusting the spine.

My clinical experience was basic in that we had to see a few hundred visits over the year in order to graduate. We also had to have a certain amount of patients have blood and urine tests taken during this time. Looking back, I really wasn't adequately prepared enough to go out on my own right after graduation day, which was in June of 1989 without taking any summers off.

I moved back to Pennsylvania and began working as an associate doctor in York, PA in an amazing, very well equipped clinic with 15 or more treatment rooms, and all kinds of therapy equipment in each room. A group of doctors did a lot of diagnostic testing such as work strength evaluations, and x-rays. This is where I came in; I was the exam doctor and took x-rays. I learned a lot from the experienced doctors, but unfortunately this is where I first realized the lure of financial gain can sometimes become more important than patient care. After 6 months of experience, I looked elsewhere for a doctor seeking to hire an associate with a buyout option and found one in Camp Hill, PA. In June of 1990, I began working with this very personable and experienced doctor, who had practiced in California in one of the biggest nutritional clinics of the time. Unfortunately, he explained more of how the monetary factor had a corrosive influence on the clinics owners. He was told that he was not "pushing hard enough" when doing muscle testing. Muscle testing must be objective when testing muscles for weakness. The theory is that when a muscle goes weak and you give the patient certain nutrition, it will become strong again if the body needs it. The problem is, however, this practice got busier and had to hire more employees resulting in a higher overhead. Thus the objectivity went out the window; the owners told him he was not selling enough vitamins.

In June of 1991, I bought this Camp hill practice and even opened up a satellite clinic for a short while in 1993. Interestingly enough, I ended up closing this satellite because the owner, an Internal medicine doctor would never refer anyone to me. His walls were paper thin and one day I heard him ask a patient how his back pain was and then he answered "Take some Advil and put some heat on it." The strange thing is, just the week before I saw him outside, and he stopped me and said, "You guys do a good service; when patients go to a physical therapist they just put some electrodes and throw a heat pack on them and charge $85. You guys do a better service" Makes you wonder?

Over the years I had several partners from 1995-1997 and with one I shared space and opened up a satellite together. I also practiced in Harrisburg and while there looked around for a small town that would be a good place to raise our daughters and found it in Mount Holly

Springs, just south of Carlisle. In 2000 I moved to my current house, twelve steps from my office, on 2.5 beautiful acres and have been here ever since.

CHAPTER THREE

Plowing Through the Years in Practice

I am working along through the years treating mostly neck and back sprains and strains with pretty impressive results. Keep in mind that Mayo clinic only gets about 33% results. Less than a few percent of patients, which I have treated over the years, did not receive any relief. I have always been mystified over the high expectations patients seem to have about a chiropractic treatment method so chided and unaccepted by conventional medicine. By this I mean that if medicine did not solve their health concern after three months of drugs and physical therapy, why expect me to get them better in one visit? Why did they not come here first instead of last? Isn't this much less invasive than drugs and surgery? This is an example of the medical model brainwashing at its finest. We were all told growing up that conventional medicine is everything and anything else is on the fringe of science, not really accepted as truth. I hope to expand your way of thinking by the end of this book.

In 2007 I decided become more specialized in the treatment of chronic disc cases so I took a certification course and bought cutting edge traction/decompression equipment. I can honestly say ever since then, my success rates with both lower back and disc cases have been incredible at >90%.

I have always thought that if I could invite medical doctors to observe what I do they would be amazed at the logical progression of thinking involved in, a disc problem case, for example. The ensuing treatment used is both comfortable and highly effective. There is no jumping off the ropes as in the World Wrestling Federation or digging my elbow on the patient's back. These are the images that most medical doctor's disapproval of chiropractic treatment conjures up. Part of me however, thinks they do not want to know the effectiveness of chiropractic treatment. If they did and still did not refer patients, wouldn't they be hypocrites? I always thought it was the outcome or the patient's best interest that is most important. Patients always tell me that the relations between the medical field and alternative doctors have gotten better over the years. I can honestly say that I hardly EVER get a referral from a medical doctor or osteopath; I can count only a few in my twenty-five years since graduation. Now **a few** patients would say that they came in to my office because their doctor told them to go to a chiropractor, but, never mentioned anyone's name.

Statistics show that chiropractors are now only seeing 7% of the population down from the 10% we were seeing in the nineties. Of those 7% over 90% had a pleasant experience and were extremely satisfied with the outcome. My frustration is with the 93% who NEVER went to a chiropractor, including those in the medical profession who CONSTANTLY badmouth us. In 2012 Big Pharma (drug companies) spent $27 billion a year in advertising to make sure the public is on a pill- for- every- ill- treadmill.

One day about two years ago, I had an epiphany that would change my professional life. Reading through my chiropractic journal, I saw an ad for a Neuro/Metabolic super group by, Dr. Mike Johnson, a chiropractic neurologist, who claimed to treat chronic patients who could not improve by using both conventional medical and chiropractic methods. He touted the idea that people will pay a fair price to those with the knowledge to get them better. He has 450 doctors in his program, which he formulated in 2007. Like me and many other chiropractors, he was not satisfied with the current results anyone in the health field was getting with chronically ill patients who had nowhere else to turn. Dr. Johnson looked deeper into the field of neurology at the Carrick Institute, which offered a postgraduate study in neurology. He completed the three year certification program and began to have incredible results with the tough chronic cases. Moreover, he generously shared his successful results with other chiropractors who asked him what his treatment model was and how he incorporated what he had learned into his practice; thus the Neuro- Super group was born. Dr. Johnson actually created a forum or board on the Internet with educational information for members on how to treat these chronic patients. Importantly, the forum also allows member doctors to correspond and exchange information. Listening to many doctor testimonials and I even called a few doctors to ask about the program, only receiving great endorsements from everyone I talked to.

About two and a half years ago, I joined this Neuro-Metabolic super group. Since then, this message board, by Dr. Johnson, developed its other half, or the metabolic side of the neurometaboliic group of doctors. I joined the group right about the time when the metabolic side took off. Many of the member doctors posted their miracle cases on the forum board. It is unbelievable that even chronic musculoskeletal (back or neck pain) pain patients were improving with metabolic or nutritional treatment. I read this statement from some of the doctor's on the board: "If you had to choose and only had one form of treatment, **metabolic (nutritional) trumps everything else**." There was a testimonial, on the board, of a post cervical disc surgery patient who did not improve until treated nutritionally. Moreover, another woman with severe digestive complaints did not recover until tested for cross reactivity with gluten (wheat protein) and found to be sensitive to rice. When she stopped eating rice, EVERY SYMPTOM she had been experiencing was gone. There were also many patients with seemingly unrelated conditions, ranging from heart problems to kidney trouble and liver dysfunction that improved when treated metabolically. Often times this treatment involves avoidance as well as only eating certain foods.

14

I was already following many of the nutritional guidelines that the members of the neurometaboliic group was advocating for one to be healthy. With the exception of going "gluten free," I was walking the talk before my talk was even happening, and was extremely excited and liberated to think my nutritional philosophy is now justified.

I realized the need to incorporate my own lifestyle and nutritional principles into my chiropractic practice. My wife had been saying for years that I should add nutrition to my practice because many of the other mothers she met, at their kids' sporting events, would question her about certain foods or vitamins.

I decided to take further nutritional courses with a goal to become a certified function medicine practitioner as well as a certified clinical nutritionist. Currently, I have the functional medicine certification and am in the process of getting started with a certification in clinical nutrition.

CHAPTER FOUR

Why Are We So Unhealthy: The American Diet

There are two main reasons why so many in the country have such poor health: ***Free radical damage*** and ***Excitotoxins***. Free radical damage occurs when a cell with an unpaired electron robs an electron from another cell making it unstable. This action goes on and on like a domino effect; the target point for the cell damage is the mitochondrial DNA or powerhouse of the cell; this DNA in the cell is ten times more susceptible to damage than the rest of the cell. **There are three main causes of free radical damage in today's society: The poor SAD (standardized American diet), heavy metal toxicity, and toxic chemicals.**

Let me add here that my wife says my explanations get too technical and I must admit that this may be one of those times; however, this is very important information.

First I will discuss the SAD. Becky read a quote to me a few days ago, that is so profound I must repeat it here. *"We are fed by the food industry which does not care at all about our health and treated by the health industry which does not care at all about our diet. "*

Since we started processing grains, the health of the country as a whole has been declining. Thus the white flour curse, part of the white death trio, along with white sugar and white salt, begins. I first heard of this white death term from Dr. Johnson. Grains turn into sugar fast; there is no getting around it. The early grains were grown in much richer soil. Most people do not realize that the soil content today has 14% of the mineral content it had in 1934, when my father was born. Thus, these grains grown in the soil rich with minerals were far healthier than the grains we ingest today on a regular basis.

Even rich soil cannot compete with the greed of the impending industrialized roller-milling revolution.

Let me do a quick explanation of the history of white flour and how it has adversely impacted our health. Before 1817 all flour was simply stone ground wheat containing 28% protein. Near the end of the eighteen hundreds, all grinding stones had been replaced with iron, steel, and porcelain rollers; thus refined flour became the first "fast food," if you will. However, before the rollers were changed, the wheat could not become entirely white. The grinding wheel removed the bran or fiber part of the wheat kernel but left the germ containing the nutritive oils intact. This germ was crushed by the stone and gave the flour a yellowish tint. These oils also shortened the shelf life of the flour which soon would turn rancid by oxidation. Now you have every grain merchant's nightmare, a grain that smells bad and goes rancid fast. Because of yellow color, the fact that any nutritional benefit was in the germ seemed to be ignored and nullified by the social stigma of eating the "yellow colored, smelly flour." The new roller milling procedure simply removed the germ, as well as the fiber, leaving nothing but a starch, void of any nutrition. This flour now looked white and would stay on the shelf long enough for people to buy it. Ironically, corn and rice flours were to meet the same fate. With the refined flours came disease from malnutrition, mostly B vitamin deficiencies. About fifty years later, vitamins were discovered and thus the treatment for those rampant diseases. The government mandated that all white flour had to have B vitamins added. Moreover, in the late 1990's, the government also made it mandatory to add folic acid as well. Today's wheat only is about 8-12% protein. Look at the results of all of this inferior grain consumption: a major contributor to the widespread obesity in this country which leads to increased diabetes, heart disease, and cancer. When you "enrich" something, you strip it of its natural vitamins and infuse it with synthetic ones. Synthetic vitamins should not be taken because the body cells resonate with a certain light frequency. I know this may sound like voodoo to you so wait until I get to the later chapters on bioenergy medicine and nutrition. The synthetic vitamins only contain minute amounts of natural substances, which fool the body cells to let them in. Then as time goes by the synthetic content of the vitamins causes bodily stress and ends up as accumulated toxins, some of which get excreted in the urine, feces or sweat if the person is lucky. If the liver and gallbladder are not in good working condition for phase one detoxification, these toxins will become bio accumulated in the liver. Let me give you a great example about how today's white flour is "enriched "with iron. Rock iron is pulverized and mixed with the white flour, however, the problem is that rock iron is an inferior junk form of iron and as it accumulates in the liver it prevents the liver from absorbing good quality iron needed to make tyrosine and adrenaline. Tyrosine is an amino acid that is needed to make the thyroid hormone T4. Could this white flour consumption have anything to do with the 30 million undiagnosed thyroid cases? Adrenaline, a hormone made by your adrenal glands, is needed to hold the mineral magnesium, needed for proper muscle function, in the blood. It releases stored energy in the muscles, is essential for bone formation, calcium absorption, and regulates body temperature. Can you now see how white flour consumption leads to a downward spiral of your overall health?

The second component of white death is white sugar. On average, each person in America eats 142 pounds a sugar per year. I have been harping on the evils of excessive sugar for years but now it seems like it finally may not be falling on deaf ears as it has for such a long time.

There are different forms of sugar; the two most popular are sucrose and high fructose corn syrup. Sucrose, or refined white sugar, is also known as table sugar. The other form of sugar is high fructose corn syrup. Chemically, the two are almost identical. Each contains half fructose and half glucose.

Every living thing on earth uses glucose for energy. If you get your fructose from its origin, in fruits and vegetables, you you would consume about 15 grams per day; this was the case a hundred years ago. Today, however, the typical adolescent gets 73 grams per day mostly from sweetened drinks containing no fiber or any nutrients. Then on the other hand, fructose from fruits and vegetables has fiber, vitamins, minerals, enzymes, and beneficial plant nutrients, all of which moderate any negative metabolic effects. In this case, fructose is not the problem but the huge amounts of it people are consuming. Also most of the calories people consume today are added sugars in the form of high fructose corn syrup (HFCS). And ironically, most of the foods people rely on to lose weight, the low-fat diet foods, are the highest in fructose. But unlike the fructose from fruit and vegetables, all of the fiber has been removed so there is no nutritive value at all. They are all, in fact, empty calories.

In fact, 55% of the sweeteners used in food processing and beverage manufacturing are made from corn. This leads to the invention of HFCS, introduced in the 1970s as a substituting in pastries because it was cheaper to manufacture and had a longer shelf life. Can anyone say TRANS FATTY ACIDS? I will talk about them later. I also recently saw a commercial where that said, "sugar is sugar" and that your body reacts to high fructose corn syrup the same way as it does sugar. This is simply NOT TRUE. The fructose in HFCS is created by having the glucose portion of it undergo several enzymatic processes to make it SWEETER. Yes, you heard this right. It is 20 times sweeter than table sugar or sucrose. The glycemic index, based on the amount of time it takes for something eaten to turn to sugar, ranges from one to 100. High fructose corn syrup has a glycemic index of 120. Yes, you read it right; it has a higher glycemic index than sugar, which has a

100% glycemic index and is what every other food is measured against. What do you think is happening with your insulin release when your body tries to get this newly consumed, sweeter than sugar food into your bloodstream? It is in overdrive. Your brain is also fooled and this makes your blood sugar spike like a jumping bean. HFCS is found mostly in soda and processed food.

Now the real danger of HFCS is the fact that it is processed differently in the liver than table sugar – as if plain white table sugar or sucrose isn't bad enough! In fact the entire burden of metabolizing fructose falls on your liver. With table sugar the liver has to break down only 20% of the glucose. Most of it is metabolized to produce energy as every cell in your body utilizes it-and then when there is extra, with the S.A.D., it gets stored as fat. The fructose, in HFCS however, is all directly metabolized into free fatty acids, the damaging form of cholesterol, and triglycerides, which get stored as FAT. In fact fructose is the most attracted to fat carbohydrate. Thus, when you eat 120 calories of fructose for example, 40 calories of it get stored as fat. Less than one calorie will get sored as fat when you eat 120 calories of glucose. HFCS can cause dangerous growths of fat cells around vital organs. Can anybody not see how Type 2 or sugar diabetes can result from eating large quantities of HFCS followed by obesity and cardiovascular disease? In an article titled, "Choose Your Sweetener Carefully" by Dr. Michael Mercola D.O. that is exactly what scientists found during a 10-week study using 16 volunteers. With those on the high level fructose diet, there were new fat cells developing around the liver, heart and digestive organs. These subjects also showed signs of food processing abnormalities linked to diabetes and heart disease. The subjects on the glucose-replacing fructose diet had no such findings. Do you see a recurring theme here on how the S.A.D. adversely affects us? The problem with eating all of this processed white sugar and high fructose corn syrup is that our bodies do not have the transporters, synergists, and essential co-factors in all tissues of the body to process both of them. Thus your brain, the most voracious user of glucose wants more; you get the cravings, eat more, have mood swings, and gain weight, a viscous cycle in a failed attempt to regulate blood sugar. The worst of the worst, aside from its causing diabetes and heart disease, is that the HFCS are also a major contributor to high blood pressure, the depletion of vitamins and minerals, cancer, arthritis, and even gout. I will explore the blood sugar topic later.

A diet high in white sugar such as the S.A.D. also can lead to glycation, a fancy word meaning a protein and a sugar molecule combine, making the protein molecule much more susceptible to the free radical damage leading to AGE'S, or advanced glycation end products. This, like white flour, adversely affects the non-essential free flowing amino acid tyrosine. In this case, however, it interferes with the way your body uses it. So again, thyroid hormones, adrenaline and magnesium production and regulation, along with and all those cellular activities they are involved in downstream, will be compromised. Furthermore, this glycation also interferes with dopamine, a pleasure neurotransmitter of the brain, important for body movement, memory, learning, sleep, and attention. Parkinson's patients are low in dopamine and display involuntary movement tremors, for example. These AGE'S are the reason people with neurodegenerative diseases and chronic health conditions should not eat foods that contain fructose or refined sugar. AGE'S damage the mitochondrial DNA of the cells, which again, is 10 times more susceptible to free radical damage. **Undoubtedly, white sugar is really not the energy booster people think; in the end it ironically saps your energy instead.**

Of course, as the truth comes out about HFCS, we cannot forget the Corn Refiners Association. Remember that commercial again, which said "sugar is sugar" and its product is "natural and safe?" As Dr.

Mercola stated "cocaine is natural too, but you would not want to eat 142 pounds of it each year." HFCS is so pervasive not only in the baked goods, and sodas, as I have previously mentioned, but also in most salad dressings, condiments, and virtually ALL processed foods. Since its invention in the 1970s and inclusion into the western diet, HFCS has been a billion dollar bonanza for the corn industry. Although, the FDA (Food and Drug Administration) classifies HFCS as GRAS (generally regarded as safe), there are TONS of information to the contrary; showing that fructose is not safe. Because the adverse effects on the nation's declining health were not immediately known, medical authorities did not see its dangers. It has taken the last thirty years to recognize the bad effects from this nutritional misinformation.

I must talk a little bit about sugary, caffeine laden drinks here. Let's discuss soda first. While writing the previous paragraph, I have been trying to understand why so many people regularly drink soda, especially a supersized one at 40 ounces. There are 10 teaspoons, or 40gms of sugar in your average 12-ounce cola; that means there are 35-40 teaspoons of sugar in these mammoth supersize sodas. HOLY COW! The NUMBER ONE source of calories in America is soda in the form of HFCS. When dealing with soft drinks we cannot ignore the phosphoric acid added to colas making them taste better. This causes an acidic pH in the body and leeches calcium out of the bones greatly increases the chances for osteoporosis. Your pH is a measure of your body's mineral content. This soda consumption shows another way how minerals are adversely impacted by the S.A.D. Phosphoric acid to calcium should be in a 1:1 ratio to be healthy. In the colas it is in a 2:1 and sometimes even a 5:1 ratio. This high acid content damages the enamel on teeth; it is even worse in kids since their teeth are more porous and more susceptible to damage. There are those who only drink "diet" soda and feel they are more beneficial than "regular" sodas. Well, I do not mean to rain on their health food/good intention kick, but they will have a harder time losing weight, drinking diet soda. Even people who drank just ONE diet soda a day are at risk for problems; diet soda is void of any nutrition. Many people over eat junk foods thinking, since they are drinking diet soda, they are saving calories to spread out throughout the day. For them, there is a 36% increase in metabolic syndrome, a precursor of diabetes. Metabolic syndrome is a combination of high blood pressure, heart disease, and high triglyceride levels. Furthermore, diet soda can also alter estrogen levels in younger women, and due to its high caffeine content can actually dehydrate you. So much for drinking soda to quench your thirst; I do not see how it is worth the risk.

With the cola sugary drinks, we cannot forget the success of Starbucks. Recently, a company CEO on the evening news responded to questions about one drink that has 80 grams of sugar and 575 calories. The news anchor said that a coke only has 50 grams of sugar and is only 265 calories, and they are blamed for being so unhealthy. The CEO responded that this sugary concoction is less than 1% of their total sales. It seems he forgot to mention the carmel, chocolate, and other sugary syrups in most of their other drinks Starbucks dispenses to millions of willing recipients.

The third "White death" component, or white salt, is highly "processed, refined, and enriched". Remember earlier how I said to watch out for ENRICHED? Well, "REFINED" is the other half of that process in which the refiners strip all of the nutrients away and; it is refined so there are no minerals left. This is the case with white salt. It is refined so there are no minerals left; the remaining two components left of white salt are sodium and chloride. Dr. David Brownstein's book titled "Salt Your Way to Health" does an excellent job in thoroughly covering this whole subject; I will only touch its surface. Let's talk about what refining the salt entails. The refining process begins with the brine, a highly concentrated solution of salt and water. Usually the minerals, referred to as "impurities", are removed with such chemicals as sulfuric acid or chlorine, known as highly toxic chemicals to the body. Iodine is added to this salt but it is not enough to counter the effects of goiter, a component of thyroid disease, that it was designed to do. These minerals are then sold to be used in various industries including the vitamin one. The liquid mixture left is exposed to intense heat to evaporate it. This heat however, damages the salt molecule. Why strip the minerals you ask? Remember the white flour history. First there is the problem of shelf life; ***anything devoid of nutrition is usually not going to spoil***. Next is the white color; like the yellow tainted flour, the natural color of salt is grayer than, and not nearly as white, as the finished refined product. The manufacturers thought the more "pure" white salt would sell much better in the aisles of the grocery stores. Finally, if the salt came from a polluted area, they figured all of the toxins would be removed with refinement. Explain that rationale to me? You are taking out anything nutritive to the body with harsh chemicals on the chance it was polluted with something? Even worse, white salt is also grated with metal plates and usually contaminated with nickel. Incidentally, many women who have trouble wearing certain jewelry have a problem with nickel. Could this have to do with their consumption of white salt? Nickel will also be a factor later when I discuss heavy metal toxicity.

The Energy drink craze is the next topic when discussing the S.A.D. It is unbelievable how many kids and adults are regularly drinking energy drinks, loaded with sugar and caffeine, throughout the day; yet, they classified in the nutritional supplement category to avoid FDA regulation. The range of caffeine in energy drinks is from 50 mg to an incredible 500mg. When it comes to the damages caffeine, especially excess caffeine, causes there is little disagreement in the medical community; in fact it can raise blood pressure, disrupt sleep habits, aggravate psychiatric conditions, and is addictive. Excessive caffeine consumption can also cause caffeine intoxication that leads to a fast heartbeat, vomiting, seizure, and in some cases even death due to heart attack. This revelation came ten months after the death of a fourteen-year-old girl who consumed two 24-ounce energy drinks within a 24-hour period. Moreover, the Substance Abuse and Mental Health Services Administration found the number of emergency room visits due to energy drinks rose tenfold between 2005 and 2009. Monster Inc., the king of the energy drinks, made a statement that they were changing their classification from a nutritional supplement to a beverage to avoid being linked to any of these emergency room visits or even deaths. They also wanted to stop any "misguided criticism that a nutritional supplement is more lightly regulated than a beverage."

As dangerous as the highly caffeinated energy drinks are, the practice of mixing Red Bull with alcohol is even more dangerous. This is "a time bomb "that "attacks the liver directly," preventing the area affected from ever being regenerated. Red Bull contains a highly dangerous chemical knows as glucuronolactone; this substance is categorized as a medical stimulant, and was used in Vietnam to boost the morale of troops. It acted like a hallucinogenic and calmed war stress. However, because its effects were so devastating to those who used it, its use was discontinued; it thinned the blood and required less activity from the heart to pump the blood increasing the risk of cerebral hemorrhage.

Another component of the S.A.D. is trans fatty acids. When you see this term you should immediately think of long shelf life and poor health effects. My wife recounted of an experiment involving a McDonald's hamburger placed on a plate next to a regular hamburger. They were presented to rats for two weeks. When they researchers came back, they found the McDonald's hamburger still untouched with no signs of spoilage. They left the hamburger there for almost a year and it still looked the same. The animals were apparently smarter than humans who frequently eat at the fast food chains; the rats quickly devoured the regular hamburger. Trans fats are made when vegetable oils are hardened into margarine or shortening. Here is another shocker for most people. Canola oil, considered healthy, is really a genetically modified food; there is no such thing as a canola plant or bean etc.... In fact, canola oil is made with by dozen chemical processes so that it can withstand high temperature cooking. The result is a product that contains 40% trans fatty acids more than soybean and other junk vegetable oils such as safflower, sunflower, and corn. I will talk in detail about these oils in a later section. Remember, they are big in pastries, cookies, crackers, donuts, fried chicken, French fries, salad dressing, and many more processed foods. These are artery cloggers that can raise the levels of the harmful cholesterol or LDL and lower the levels of the good cholesterol or HDL lead to harmful diseases like type 2 diabetes. The Federal Register explained that in 1985 the FDA knew about the terrible effects of canola oil and outlawed its use in baby formula because it RETARTED GROWTH. Why all of a sudden, 28 years later, is canola oil good for everyone else? We know that Harvard researchers at the school of public health deemed trans-fats are not safe at any levels; yet food manufacturers are allowed, by the FDA, to label foods "NO TRANS FATS" as long as the product contains less than 500 mg of trans fats per ½ cup.

The S.A.D. causes various food sensitivities to dairy, soy, and the most importantly gluten that are adversely affecting so very many people. Dairy, soy, and wheat gluten are delicate subjects because there are so many people benefiting financially from them. Because I sometimes have patients who are first, second, and third generation farmers, I must be very careful about discussing the dangers of their crops because this is their livelihood.

Cow's milk, cheese and butter, including eggs which are not classified as dairy, are among the chief causes of food sensitivities; in fact they cause 85% of them. I want to focus on the effects of cow's milk on humans. This food is the perfect food for calves until they are weaned, just as breast milk is for humans. We are the only creatures, however, who continue to drink species milk beyond the weaning period. In alternative medicine, there is much discussion about the dairy industry myth. Here are some truths of cow's milk that most people do not know. Cow's milk is meant to get calves to 1000-1200 pounds in a year or so and contains many active hormones and scores of allergens in it. And alarming, has measurable quantities of toxic chemicals such as pesticides, herbicides, blood, feces, bacteria, viruses, and up to fifty antibiotics. Anything the cows eat is obviously in their milk; some cow's milk has even been found to have traces of radioactive fallout from nuke testing. There is strong epidemiological evidence that feeding cow's milk to infants has a propensity leading to iron deficiency and dehydration.

The digestive complaints people describe after drinking milk are from digesting its' sugar or lactose. It usually results in bloating, diarrhea, and abdominal cramps. Most importantly, many humans are highly allergic to cow's milk. Kids with recurrent ear infections were twice as likely to suffer from this allergy.

Recently, I saw a poster from www.notmilk.com that stated one glass of milk is allowed legally to have 135 pus cells in it! That does not sound too appetizing does it? It continued to state that the main protein in milk "casein," is toxic to humans, causing a list of symptoms such as: eczema, acne, kidney disease, arthritis, tooth decay, irritable bowel, sinus problems, colitis, Crohn's, and multiple sclerosis. Keep in mind that all of this information is interrelated to other systems in the body; this is really a list of many autoimmune diseases with many dietary causes.

More alarming facts, on cow's milk, were posted on our forum by Dr. Lonnie Herman in May of 2013 on the Johnson Forum. Dr. Herman stated many cows actually carry a bovine leukemia, which can be passed on to their offspring in their milk. It is interesting to note that the big milk producing states have much higher rates of human leukemia.

Johnne's disease is also passed on to a cow's offspring. Its symptoms are just like Crohn's disease: the cramping, gas, gut lesions, colon abscesses, and uncontrollable diarrhea. It is estimated that 60% of the population of Wisconsin, a huge milk producer, would test positive for Johnne's disease. This makes one ask the question, how many humans have contracted Crohn's from infected cows?

The one fact that makes perfect sense; the hormone IGF 1 or insulin growth factor, occurring naturally cow's milk gets a calf up to 1000-1200 pounds in one year. This EXACTLY mimics the IGF 1 in humans. When humans drink this cow's milk, the cow's IGF 1 causes our bodies to move sugars into the cells faster than we normally would increasing the chances for obesity and metabolic syndrome. Thus we may have metabolic syndrome, which then leads to diabetes. And when a cow receives additional Bovine Growth Hormone, that IGF becomes magnified by 80%; therefore we are consuming too much IGF 1. This magnifies even more the predisposition for obesity and eventually diabetes. In essence drinking cow's milk is making many people sick.

I will briefly mention cheese here which takes a lot of milk to make; in fact, a factor of 10 times more. So do not forget about cheese when you are considering milk and dairy allergies. The center for disease control says that children are taking longer to outgrow milk allergies than at any other time in history. One in 50 kids will develop a milk and egg allergy at some point in their lives.

There are literally thousands of studies on unfermented soy, the harmful soy that Americans consume. When processing soy in the western world, the soybean is separated into two golden products:

protein and oil, neither of which is safe or natural when eaten by humans. Ingestion of this soy has been linked to various diseases. In a book called "The Whole Soy Story," by Dr. Kayla Daniel, thousands of studies are described showing a cause and effect relationship between soy and digestive problems, immune distress, thyroid problems, mental decline, infertility, even cancer and heart disease.

A recent article by Dr. Mercola explains how ninety percent of the soy in this country is GMO, or genetically modified because growers want the soy to become resistant to Roundup, a toxic weed killer, in order to maximize crop yields at the cheapest price. The GMO soy also contains a bacterium that is new to our food supply. Moreover, the gene inserted into the GMO soy has been verified in a study to get into the cell DNA and continue to function. This means long after it is eaten, it can keep producing allergic proteins in your intestines. Russian studies have shown that there is even a potential for infertility in future generations. There are also "anti-nutritional factors" which include saponins, soyatoxin, phylates, protein inhibitors, oxalates, goitrogens, and estrogens. Some of these factors interfere with the enzymes you need to digest protein. This would really not really be a factor, however, if only a small amount was consumed. America's soy consumption is extremely high; about 80% of the world's soy is used in animal feed.

Fermented soy, used only as a condiment, one or two tablespoons on average, is the soy consumed in Asia. The form of soy that is nutritious has to be organic and fermented; tofu is non-fermented soy and should be avoided.

Today we have far too many harmful GMO foods. Genetically modified organisms are those in which the genetic material (DNA) has been adversely altered; GMO is also known as "genetic engineering," "biotechnology", or "recombinant DNA technology." It consists of randomly inserting genetic material-fragments of DNA, from one organism to another, usually from different species. Gluten is often modified with E coli, harmful bacteria which are the most popular carrier of DNA from organism to organism. Shortly, I will talk about aspartame, which is the "excitotoxin" found in NutraSweet. Guess how it is made? Aspartame is literally the fecal matter (poop) of genetically engineered E. coli. Producers feed these bacteria toxic waste and they defecate (poop) aspartame. Needless to say, I was blown away by that discovery! Today's gluten is also preserved with formaldehyde, a known carcinogen. Natural breeding processes have been used safely for several hundred years. Genetic engineering crop technology, however, has only been used commercially for about 10 years or so. Several early animal studies show specific disease processes resulting from genetic engineering such as: infertility, immune dysregulation, accelerated aging, abnormal gene regulation associated with cholesterol synthesis, and changes in the liver, kidney, spleen, and gastrointestinal system. Because of the mounting data, those critical of the biotechnology industry i.e., The American Academy of Environmental Medicine, maintains it is biologically plausible that genetically modified foods cause adverse health effects in humans. It is well known in the field of epigenetics that if you alter a lab rat for instance, the rat will pass this trait on to future generations due to the altered DNA. We have genetically modified, formaldehyde laced gluten that has been added to our diet for years. Do you see where I am going with this and the gluten epidemic? This should be very obvious to everyone. You cannot mess with Mother Nature and come away unscathed. One critic of the GMO corporations put it right when he said producers should just put a skull and cross bones on the packaging of all GMO foods because of the long-term health risks.

A few weeks ago, I saw a news show on the cloning of salmon. The newsman reported that the cloned or GM (genetically modified) salmon are all female and contain three chromosomes instead of the usual two, and are also 50% larger than the salmon Mother Nature produces. They grow twice as fast because of their being given a growth hormone from Pacific Chinook salmon, as well as a gene from an eel-like fish called an ocean pout. This gene acts like a switch to turn the growth hormone on all year whereas in the natural salmon it is only on for part of the year. In an experiment, the newscaster sat down to a meal prepared with both types of salmon. Surprisingly, he could not tell any difference in taste or texture between them. The problem is, however, that our bodies do not accept or recognize GMO substances as natural; therefore the autoimmune reaction in which your body attacks itself occurs as a case of mistaken identity. Another problem, according to a recent report, is that food manufacturers do not wish to be responsible for labeling whether this salmon is natural or GMO salmon. Frankenfish is the name given by opponents to the GMO salmon. AquaBounty, the company behind the GMO salmon, states that their fish "are all sterile and grown in secure containers on land-based fish farms". They did admit, however, that some fish might still be able to breed. GM Free, an anti GMO company argues that "the sterility system does not guarantee that there will not be escapees into the wild and that some of them will be fully fertile." What a disaster that could be. It may not be long now until the natural salmon will no longer exist and this GMO version will breed with the natural one; the "wild caught" salmon may become a thing of the past. Remember what happened and continues to happen with many crops. The New Animal Drug Application, the FDA Draft unfortunately agrees with AquaBounty that the salmon escaping and breeding is "extremely unlikely", and that the fish will not have any significant impacts on the quality of the environment of the United States. However, keep in mind, their monetary incentive clouds objectivity so that they turn a blind eye rather than admit the potential consequences of their ACTIONS, greatly contributing to the already unhealthy American diet?

I recently read a blurb that came up on an e-mail: Former head of Monsanto to work for the FDA. Monsanto is one of the largest, if not the largest GMO food corps today. Can everyone reading this, repeat after me: BIASED decision making. The way it stands, the FDA maintain that the GMO salmon is no different at all from the wild one and, therefore, are giving it their seal of approval. All that stands in the way of the GMO salmon being distributed to our dinner plates and restaurants are the objections from the health conscious groups who oppose all GMO animal products. We are all aware, once again, that excessive financial gain overrules food logic.

Let's now discuss GMO corn. There are seven types of corn for example, grown with pesticides (like soy and wheat), which continue to develop in the DNA cells of those who consume them. Nearly all corn syrup is made from genetically modified corn.

Dr. Walter Crooks, who is a certified clinical nutritionist and a chiropractic neurologist, developed a chart comparing the poison and nutrient content of corn and GMO corn listed in ppm (parts per million). First are the poisons in the GMO corn:

formaldehyde- 200 ppm
glyphosate- 13ppm
chemical content- 60 ppm

The organic corn has <u>zero</u> in all three categories. Here are the nutrient content in GMO corn also listed in ppm:

phosphate- 3ppm
postasium-7 ppm
calcium-14 ppm
magnesium- 2ppm
sodium-2ppm
manganese-2ppm
iron-2ppm

zinc-2.3ppm
copper-2.6ppm
cobalt-.2ppm
molybdenum- .2ppm
boron-.2ppm.

Here the nutrients in organic corn:

phosphate- 44ppm
potassium- 113ppm
calcium- 6130 ppm
magnesium- 113ppm
sodium- 0.2ppm
manganese -14ppm
iron- 14.3ppm
zinc -14.3ppm
copper -16ppm
cobalt- 1.5 ppm
molybdenum -1.5ppm
boron – 1.5 ppm

This comparison enables you to see the high nutritional content in organic corn versus the poisons, and inadequate minerals in the non-nutritive GMO corn. Our bodies have certain immune cells that police what gets into them and determine if it is harmful or not. There are certain immune cells that tag entering foreign bodies and other immune cells that destroy them; thus there is a T1 and T2 component to our immune system. Thus, when one of these gets out of balance the immune system will run out of control and often attack itself. I will return to this component of our immune system a few times throughout this book since it is so important.

GMO wheat grains have been shown to be a causative factor in auto-immune conditions in which a person's body attacks itself in a case of mistaken identity. For example "Hashimotos," an autoimmune disease named after the Japanese doctor who discovered it in 1912, is an example of the body inadvertently attacking the thyroid gland. Since then, it has been discovered that when a person afflicted with this auto immune thyroid disease eats gluten, or the wheat protein found in wheat, barley, and rye, the immune the system attacks the thyroid gland. Significantly, the wheat today has almost the same molecular structure as the thyroid gland. Keep in mind, however, that it could be any gland that the body attacks in an autoimmune reaction. Rheumatoid arthritis occurs when the body attacks its joints. The gluten molecule also closely resembles cartilage. Multiple sclerosis is an autoimmune disease where the body attacks the myelin sheath, or the covering of nerves that transmits impulses. Diabetes is also an autoimmune reaction when the body attacks the pancreas. In Celiac's disease is when the body attacks the small intestine. I am sure you get the idea. The mechanism of how the autoimmunity begins is coined "Leaky Gut Syndrome". This is another catch phrase of recent years, although not nearly as familiar with the general public as the gluten free one. Large proteins leak into the bloodstream due to the spaces between the cells of the gut that should have remained tight. Because of ingested chemicals, antibiotics, NSAIDS, antacids, chemotherapeutic drugs, steroid drugs, birth control pills, and gluten laden foods, they have become loose. This allows larger protein molecules to enter the bloodstream which fires up the immune system to start attacking; this is where things go awry, and the body attacks itself.

At this point I am sure many of you are asking what about this "gluten free" hype? It seems to be a ubiquitous phrase which recently has erupted on the scene. In my professional opinion, this is a HUGE problem. My friends and family get sick of hearing me say it but gluten consumption is a major trigger with auto-immune reactions that I just described above. It is definitely not a fad!

Since there is so much confusion surrounding eating gluten free, I will try to show how detrimental gluten is, especially for those with an auto-immune disease. When you fully understand the seriousness of this gluten issue, you can educate those around you when the topic arises. **This is a life changer.**

When you eat gluten, it is broken down by an enzyme in your intestines called tissue transglutaminase, which makes it small enough to be absorbed in the digestive tract. The result is called deaminated gliadin and it is used in most processed foods to help bind them; hence gluten is like the glue that holds ingredients together, inexpensive "glue," at that. This makes it easier to cook with, however what is even scarier is that this deaminated gliadin is used for long term shelf life and is the reason why so many foods have long expiration dates like trans-fats. The more processed the food, usually the cheaper it is; this then parlays into a higher deaminated gliadin content. I am going to summarize the leaky gut and autoimmune in the last section of this book so that you'll really get it.

Of course there is a genetic predisposition involved in gluten and Celiac's disease. It is widely believed that those who react to gluten have a genetic predisposition; human leukocyte antigen DQ2 and HLA-DQ8 are the genes that are found in a diagnosis of Celiac's disease. Although the estimates of those in the United States with Celiac's are only 2-4% of the population, it is also estimated that 35-50% of the population has the HLA-DQ2 or DQ8 gene. So, everyone who is reading this repeat after me: "Celiac's disease in this country is hugely underestimated."

There are different classifications of how gluten affects individuals. The first is food allergies, whereby you have an immediate IGE mediated immune response which can be life threatening; your throat could close up. This is the infamous peanut or shellfish allergy we have all heard of. Secondly, there are also food reactions, in which there are some symptoms but usually not severe and not immediate. Symptoms here could occur between two hours and last up to two days after gluten is consumed. A stomach ache or nausea would be a good example. Lastly, there is a food sensitivity in which the immune system in not involved and the symptoms may seem unrelated such as a headache.

There is also enteropathy, a big word meaning disease of the intestines. In this case it refers to the villi cells on the border of the small intestine. To be definitively diagnosed with Celiac's most believe you need an actual biopsy of the small intestine. These villi cells will show pathology or disease in someone with Celiac's. New research however shows that you can actually have non celiac gluten enteropathy (diseased intestines). You can have no HLA DQ2 or DQ8 genes present and still have the diseased intestines. Here is the kicker. Only 1/3 of patients with gluten sensitivity have disease of the intestinal tract or enteropathy. This means there are 2/3 of the populations that have NO intestinal destruction or symptoms. Can anybody believe there is "silent Celiac's disease?" The British Medical Journal stated in 1999 that 87.5% of those with both a genotype (had the HLA-DQ2 or DQ8) and a positive biopsy for enteropathy had no symptoms. This leaves only 12.5% of diagnosed Celiac's patients having symptoms. The journal of Gastroenterology, in 2001, said that for every one person diagnosed with Celiac's disease with symptoms, there are eight unconfirmed cases or those with Celiac's without any gastroenterology symptoms. In the past fifty years the incidence of Celiac's was believed to be one in 700. Today's statistics show one in 100 has the disease. The greatest mortalities have been shown to be among those who have silent Celiac's disease that causes malignancies. This is probably due to their throwing caution to the wind, so to speak, with gluten consumption sine they have no idea they are afflicted with Celiac's disease. In other words, while many people lack any obvious or detectable symptoms, they are unintentionally harming themselves by consuming gluten.

Many times a patient will say, "I was checked for Celiac's disease and the doctor said it was negative and I don't have it". I tell them it is probably because most medical doctors only check one aspect of gluten, transglutaminase or alpha gliadin antibodies. There are at least 12 other components of gluten that are left unchecked. There is a lab called Cyrex which has an "array" (test) that checks for all of the components of wheat; it costs about $325. Their website is www.cyrexlabs.com.

I must mention cross reactivity. Cyrex also has a test called an array #4 for $225 to check this. The problem is that many foods have a similar amino acid sequence as gluten. Your body then makes antibodies against them. The next time you consume that food, you can experience symptoms or effects similar to those you experience when you eat gluten. In other words cross reactive foods trigger an auto-immune reaction as a case of mistaken identity.

Here is the list of cross reactive foods with gluten; cow's milk (casein), caseomorphin, milk butyrophin, American cheese, milk chocolate (dark chocolate is fine because it is the milk in the chocolate that is the problem), rye, barley, spelt, Kamut (polish wheat), yeast, oats, and coffee.

Next we have eleven foods that are not cross reactive; however, those on a gluten free diet often still seem to be sensitive to: sesame, hemp, buckwheat, sorghum, millet, amaranth, quinoa, tapioca, corn, rice, and potato (does not include sweet potatoes).

There are those that maintain, "I don't have Celiac's disease so I can eat what I want". Listen to Dr. Williams, a cardiologist, and author of the book "Wheat Belly" whose thesis is that today's wheat is "the perfect poison." In a CBS interview he explained that modern day wheat is an 18-inch tall plant born of genetic research from the 60's and 70's containing a new protein called gliadin. When eaten, gluten is broken down into gliadin and glutenin. Gliadin is then broken down into alpha, beta, gamma, and omega. He adds that he is not only addressing the celiac or wheat sensitivity sufferers, but everybody else, because "everybody else is susceptible to the gliadin protein that is an opiate." This protein binds to opiate receptors in your brain and in some people stimulates appetite, to such an extent, that one can consume an average of 440 more calories per day." Interesting, don't you agree?

"Identifying and Conquering Gluten Sensitivity inside & Outside the Gut," a CD series (compact disc) by Dr. Tom O'Brian, sited recently in the British Medical Journal, stated that every woman with osteoporosis should be tested for both gluten sensitivity and Celiac's disease. Dr. O'Brian also quoted, in the Journal of Neurology, Neurosurgery, and Psychiatry, "There is a misrepresentation that Celiac's disease only affects the intestines. Lactose intolerance, where you cannot digest lactose found in dairy products because you lack the lactase enzyme, and infertility may also be manifestations of Celiac's". He added that most people can eat oats, but often they are contaminated with gluten from processing and common shipping vehicles.

The Journal Lancelet describes a study of 1,072 Celiac disease patients who were followed for twenty-five years. At any point in their lives, the CD (Celiac disease) patients were twice as likely to die from any cause compared to their non-CD siblings- defined as a standard mortality rate of 2:1. Compliance with a gluten free diet lowered the mortality rate to .5:1 for CD patients to non-celiac patients. In other words, people with Celiac disease went from twice as likely, to half as likely upon going gluten free. Non-compliance (defined as having gluten once monthly) increased the mortality rate to 6:1 for CD patients to non- CD patients. One should consider testing for gluten sensitivity when meds for anxiety and depression do not work. Fifty percent of kids with drug resistant epilepsy were cured on a gluten free diet. There is a 320% increase of schizophrenia in those diagnosed with Celiac's disease. CD affects adults more than kids as 25% of those diagnosed are over 65 years of age; this makes sense, because they had more time to eat the S.A.D and be exposed to all the environmental toxins. There was also a decreased brain perfusion of at least one area in brain scans of CD patients in 73% of those scanned. After being treated with a GF (gluten free) diet, only one patient showed a decreased perfusion. This also involved the frontal lobe of the brain. Anxiety and depression were present in 67% of non-treated CD patients. Furthermore, ADHD can primarily be caused by CD.

With a diagnosis of CD and gluten sensitivity there is usually a familial history of either a parent or sibling having the same thing. There are GI (gluten intolerance) symptoms that most people are aware of; however, there are also neurological symptoms that most people are not such as headache and peripheral neuropathy with pins and needles in the hands and feet that diabetics often suffer from. There are also muscular symptoms; gluten sensitivity is the most common cause of myopathy or muscle pain in those over 50, next to statins that is. How many patients are coming to my office with muscle pain and overall body aches who think they have chronic fatigue syndrome and fibromyalgia? In addition, there are also long-term progressive, symmetrical muscle weakness and shrinkage known as atrophy. Developmental symptoms involved include: failure to thrive, anorexia, short stature, delayed puberty, chronic fatigue/lethargy, auto immune thyroid, osteoporosis, nose bleeds or bleeding gums.

Here are some physical signs which may indicate CD or GS: transverse white lines on teeth and fingernails, black and blue bruising easily, lymph node enlargement, altered craniofacial development in which a person's forehead has a greater vertical or north south dimension than the distance between the bottoms of their chin to the bottom of the nose.

To summarize: biopsy is no longer the gold standard to diagnose CD because it only shows end stage CD. Over 90% of CD patients have HLADQ2 and 10% have HLADQ8. Some have both, one from each parent; if you have either, you have greater risk. Certain antibodies are present in only 30-40% of the population who are GS; therefore, all 14 different antibodies should be tested by Cyrex Labs. However, the Gold Standard test for GS is a 3 month modified elimination diet. I will discuss gluten in a more practical way in the treatment section of this book. Get Dr. O'Bryan's CD set; they really go into detail.

Related to gluten is the "meat glue" problem. Apparently, restaurants use this substance, an enzyme made from the blood plasma of pigs and cows. This is dehydrated into a white powder. According to Dr. Mercola, "When then sprinkled on a protein, such as beef, it forms cross-linked, insoluble protein polymers that essentially act like super-glue, binding the pieces together with nearly invisible seams". In an accompanying video he showed this being made. Chefs take chicken or beef scraps or pieces of meat that are not in breast or roast form, sprinkle some meat glue powder on them, wrap them in clear plastic, and refrigerate them for an hour. Even butchers could not tell the difference between this concoction and solid chunks of meat. How many people eating this "gluten glue" end up sick and nobody knows why?

We also have something "pink slime" whenever we eat ground beef from the grocery store and at any fast food places. This substance is composed of the trimmings of meat ground into a fine, thick protein paste, then subject to ammonia gas to remove the bacteria. When restaurants and grocery stores buy this ground meat, they never know where this meat comes from; you can have a burger from many different cows and even from different countries! The use of ammonia in this protein paste process robs the body of nucleotides which makes up cells. We need 6 billion of them to make up one cell. The ammonia interferes with this process making it harder for your body to turn over new cells and therefore makes you age faster. Significantly, other foods containing ammonia are Chips Ahoy cookies, Velveeta cheese, Wonder bread, Chef Boyardee ravioli, and some cocoa brands.

I will add this chapter on the S.A.D. with a brief discussion about the importance of water consumption. Most Americans are chronically partially dehydrated. I constantly hear patients tell me they do not like or even HATE water. Yes, you read it right. Many say they do not drink any plain water, saying they get it in their coffee, tea, sports drink, and soda and ask me if that is good enough. Think about the job your kidneys have to do; in the course of a day they must filter 2000 liters of blood. When you do not drink enough water, your kidneys and your adrenal glands will not function properly. All of the drinks I mentioned above, with the addition of alcohol, cause dehydration; Dr. Marshall from Premiere Research Labs, states that an eight-ounce cup of coffee will nullify thirty-two ounces of water due to its dehydration property. With all of these caffeinated beverages consumed on a daily basis, for example, most Americans are chronically partially dehydrated. There is no substitute for PLAIN water; it is essential for good health. Most tap water is loaded with fluoride and chlorine, toxic to our bodies, and competing with iodine molecule in the thyroid. This gland is the "spark plug" for energy. This iodine is needed to make thyroid hormones. I will get into more on this in the last section of the book.

CHAPTER FIVE

Why Are We So Unhealthy: The Toxic Brew

The second factor contributing to free radical damage is exposure and consumption of *toxic chemicals*. I want to mention vaccinations because they contain heavy doses of toxic chemicals, such as mercury, administered almost at birth and continued throughout adolescence. This is a highly controversial topic, which continues to be researched and discussed. Each of you should become familiar with both sides of the argument.

Dr. Mercola interviewed Dr. Andrew Wakefield, a pediatric surgeon/researcher, who has had over 100 peer review papers published. With one study he performed and submitted to the "Lancelet", a very prestigious medical journal, in 2008, he found a connection between the measles virus, digestive problems, and learning disorders. Upon further investigation, he actually found a link between MMR (measles, mumps, and rubella) vaccine and autism. This was in 2008 but in 2010 he was forced to retract his study's findings as "unfounded" and flawed. The British council investigating his findings said nobody could replicate them. Arguably, it also points out the lengths the medical field will go to in order to squash research that does not support its bottom line.

In another article on the internet on November 13, 2013, by Dr. Diane Harper lead researcher for the HPV vaccine Gardasil, she made the astonishing admission that the Gardasil vaccine is a "huge deadly scam." The article was removed shortly thereafter. Makes you wonder who was watching. Keep in mind, the vaccination industry is a multibillion dollar industry and its ceo's are not going to tolerate naysayers who question their effectiveness or safety.

There are over 80,000 toxic chemicals commercially produced in the United States today. Many of these were developed after World War II, and not surprisingly, the long-term use and effects of many of these have never been adequately investigated. Furthermore, the term "low dose" is very misleading, implying that all low concentrations are harmless. As you may have thought, many of these chemicals are extremely harmful in very low doses. For example, the herbicide 2, 4 5T is harmful in parts per trillion; no chemical herbicides are without dangerous side effects. I have had many patients over the years tell me that they regularly get their liver enzymes checked because of the long-term use of a statins or anti-inflammatory drugs. Their medical doctor always tells them that they are "within safe levels." Unless they are generated by the body, the body's level of chemicals should be non-detectable and not "low level." I always said there really are no safe levels. Your liver will suffer from having to process these statin drugs. Is the risk worth the benefit?

Perhaps one of the most insidious examples of this is fluoridation of the water supply. There is a shocking new documentary called, "Flouridegate", which is a real eye opener that you can order on the internet on flouridegate.org. It explains the government knows of the harmful effects of fluoridated water, especially in young children, and yet they fight to protect the policies enforcing it. In the early 1950's and 1960's the Office of the Public Health Service were at the heart of the pro-fluoride push. The US Public Health Service and the New York Health State Department - which is of course, heavily subsidized by the P.H.S. - had representatives who supported fluoridation in a booklet called "Our Children's Teeth." Ironically, a group called the Committee to Protect Our Children's Teeth put out this booklet. To these representatives fluoridation meant money, jobs, and power. The National Academy of Sciences and Harvard, is also heavily subsidized by the P.H.S., also made favorable comments in this publication. Harvard received $7 million in research grants in 1960 from P.H.S. The A.D.A. (American Dental Association) also received $78,000 in 1958 and 108,000 in 1960 from. Most people know that the A.D.A is the most fervent supporter of fluoridation.

Here is what we do know about fluoride, however. Two new studies from previously classified government research confirms the neurotoxic effects of fluoride on the human brain and showed children exposed to higher levels of fluoride had lower IQ's. Notable, well known medical doctors are advocating extremely low doses, only drops on a tooth brush of those fewer than six years of age. There have been many acute poisoning cases prompting a poison warning on the label of all fluoridated toothpastes sold in the United States; in fact, a 7 ounce tube of toothpaste contains 199 mg of fluoride which would be fatal if ingested!

Moreover, a large and increasing number of children are succumbing to dental fluorosis, which is permanent adverse structural damage to the teeth. Animal studies revealed ADD-like symptoms in offspring of pregnant females exposed to relatively low doses. Young and adult animals exposed to fluoride experienced the opposite effect-sluggishness or hypoactivity. One study published in "Brain Research" showed that drinking only 1 part per million Fluoride (NaF) in water had histologic lesions in the brain similar to neurodegenerative diseases such as Alzheimer's or dementia.

Fluoride is also carcinogenic. The Department of Health of New Jersey found that bone cancer in male children occurred at a two to seven time's greater rate with those living in a fluoridated area. The EPA (Environmental Protection Agency) confirmed bone cancer causing effects of fluoride at low levels in animal studies.

It was also found that toxic levels of fluoride build up in the bones thus weakening their tensile strength leading to an increase in hip fractures. Hip fractures are a huge problem in this country with the elderly.

Independent Research has shown that immune system disorders are steadily increasing in the generation exposed to the toxic fluoridation since the 1960s and 1970s. Fluoride used to be the treatment for hyperthyroidism, in the early to mid-1900s, because it suppressed thyroid function. Fluoridation is banned in many industrialized countries. Each of us must make his own decision on fluoridation safety after investigating the most recent research available.

Another toxic chemical in the water supply, from corn crops, is atrazine. In fact, it is used on most corn crops in this country. This is an herbicide that has been shown to transform male frogs to fully fertile female frogs, and is linked to breast tumors, and prostate problems.

Many toxic chemicals are used in building construction and furniture manufacturing. The buildings of today are closed structures with few windows, allowing only a small amount of fresh air circulation; this toxic construction began in the 1980's in which indoor air pollution often exceeds the outdoor one. In fact only 40% of indoor chemicals come from outdoors, and 60% of indoor chemicals are generated by products and machines used indoors. Who is at risk for this? The exact number of those suffering from this multiple chemical sensitivity is unclear. The fact that there has been a huge rise in asthma, chronic fatigue syndrome, attention deficit disorder, and second hand smoke lung disease, are proof of these chemical's adverse effects. Chemicals are so rampant in our environment that a study done on 24,000 students at Northern Texas University found only 25 tested normal for chemical toxicity (0.1%). The ratio of females to males presenting for medical treatment is 7:1. Males usually present with more advanced disease.

The main mechanism for chemical sensitivity is failure of the body's detoxification pathways to adequately clear toxic chemicals. This is headed by the liver. Again I refer to the assault on the liver by white flour. Because most of the toxic chemicals are lipophilic, attracted to fat, they become stored in the body's fat, resistant to the body's metabolism and excretion. In fact sometimes biopsies show a 300% increase in chemicals than in circulating serum levels. Remember 1 in 3 adults are considered obese today. How toxic does that make one third of the adult population?

Cigarettes and alcohol can be sold legally but their continued use can harm and even kill you over time. Currently about one in five or 20% of Americans smoke cigarettes; they are the highest cause of preventable death in the US according to the CDC. Cigarette use in this country has really been declining over the past years, yet it still accounted for 443,000 or one in EVERY FIVE DEATHS last year. Moreover, there are 50,000 deaths per year from second hand smoke. Smoking related diseases cause the United States more than $150 billion per year. There are 445 new lung cancer cases diagnosed each day. Cigarette smoke contains over 4,000 chemicals, 50 of which are known carcinogenic or cancer causing and many are poisonous. Here is a list of the most recognizable ones: butane in lighter fluid, cadmium in batteries, stearic acid in candle wax, hexamine in barbeque lighter, toluene, part of the toxic trio, ammonia in toilet cleaner, arsenic in rat poison, and the big one, nicotine, also an insecticide. Perchlorate is a chemical found in explosives and an ingredient in rocket fuel. Research found that it contaminates our produce and gets into the water supply. The real shocker is, however, that when the perchlorate in the tobacco plant is combined with the chemical thiocyanate in tobacco smoke, it can adversely affect the thyroid gland. This was found to occur at common levels of perchlorate exposure.

Tobacco kills up to half of its regular users; in the 20th century, it killed 100 million people. Nicotine reaches your brain in ten seconds after smoke is inhaled and has been found in every part of the body and in breast milk. Cigarettes are comprised of 20% processed sugar, and many diabetics are unaware of this secret sugar intake. Moreover, there is the effect of burning the sugar which is currently unknown. "Lite" cigarettes are made by putting carbon dioxide in tobacco and then superheating it until it puffs up like expanding foam. This expanded tobacco then fills the same paper as the "regular tobacco." On average, smokers draw harder on "lite" and menthol cigarettes than on regular ones, ironically, giving them the same levels of nicotine and tar as a result. Several active ingredients and general methods of production are involved in making sure the nicotine in a cigarette is many more times potent than that of a tobacco plant. I will end this topic by noting that current research shows that if you smoke more than one pack of cigarettes per day, there is an **85%** chance that it will get you in the end. What a gloomy topic, sorry to be so pessimistic but due to the second hand smoke dangers, this topic really affects everyone.

Excessive alcohol consumption leads to free radical damage. Some studies show that when broken down in the body, the resultant chemicals cause damage similar to radiation poisoning. We also cannot forget that alcohol eventually gets broken down to sugar and therefore increases blood sugar levels. So diabetes and heart disease are a possibility. Excess alcohol consumption also lowers a male's testosterone levels. Normally, the liver produces about one ounce of alcohol per day to perform its normal routine. So alcohol warnings are addressed especially to heavier drinkers and much less to the social, one to two drinks per day crowd.

Again, a lot of this information will overlap. You previously read about the dangers of dairy tainted with pesticides, herbicides, and hormones. If the beef is not grass fed and the veggies and fruits not organic, they definitely have these substances in them. Just think about the following statistic: 70% of the antibiotics used in this country are given to animals for growth enhancement. How can this not be contributing to the early onset of puberty of our younger generation? Furthermore, this excessive use of antibiotics is primarily responsible for a rampant increase in the antibiotic resistance diseases in humans.

We consider the problems with mass food production. Many people choose not to think about this but it is a factor in why so many of us are unhealthy. Concentrated Animal Feeding Operations (CAFO) produces beef significantly different from organic grass fed beef. There are major differences in both contamination and nutritional content. The CAFO animals have a tendency to get sicker which means pathogenic contamination when you take them out of their natural environment. Just look at the USDA meat recalls for 2011 and 2012. CAFO cows are also fed GMO grains which make it even worse. Their natural diet SHOULD be grass. When they eat grains their stomachs reach a certain acidity level that is very conducive to E. coli bacteria proliferation. On the other hand, the cows eating plain grass are much less susceptible to these pathogenic organisms; organic beef contamination with E Coli is very rare. In this country it is very unfortunate that there is no federal requirement for meat grinders to test their ingredients for E. coli. In 2008 the USDA issued a voluntary guideline for meat processers to test their ingredients before grinding, but it was met with resistance from the meat industry. To matters worse, don't look for most retailers to test their products either.

Furthermore, all of this technology enabling us to feed everybody has its pitfalls. You would think that food processing should be even safer with this technology, but that is not the case. As in politics, there are too many monetary interests riding on certain inspections. Some maintain that eating in the US processed food system is like playing a game of Russian roulette.

Thus, a major problem in the US right now is food poisoning. The CDC (Centers for Disease Control) estimates anywhere between 6 to 81 million Americans contract food borne illnesses each year and food poisoning claims up to 9,000 lives annually. Considering the fact that our current food system encourages pathogens and contaminations of all kinds, it's not all that surprising that as many as one in four people get sickened each year. Most people just assume that they have a flu bug and do not even suspect food poisoning.

There is a letter posted on the Farm Freedom Alliance website by Dr. Huber, a professor at Purdue University. He wrote to Tom Vilsack, the Secretary of Agriculture, explaining that there is a pathogen found in Roundup ready GMO soybean and corn, only visible under an electron microscope on 36,000x (magnification). It is a micro fungal-like organism and is able to reproduce. He said there "is strong evidence that it promotes disease in plants and animals." Tests performed confirmed its presence in livestock and showed a high rate of spontaneous abortions and infertility; this has been escalating in frequency over the past few years and could explain the recent reports of 20% infertility rates in dairy heifers and the 45% spontaneous abortions rates in dairy cattle. This SHOULD be a worry to you if you consume these products. The WCRF (World Cancer Research Fund) reviewed more than 7,000 clinical studies, which studied the relationship between diet and cancer. They found that the preservatives in meat are a major problem. Most notable are the nitrates; you probably heard about this years ago with bacon labeled as the worst of the bunch. You must also be aware, however, of ham, some sausages, salami, peperoni, hamburgers, and hot dogs. Nitrates are not only added as preservatives, but as a coloring and flavoring agents. They are converted to nitrosamines. Sodium nitrate is added to the meat so the organism that causes BOTULISM does not develop. Nitrates are known carcinogens. The WCRF found that by just eating 1.8 ounces of processed meat daily, about one piece of sausage or three pieces of bacon, raises your cancer rate chances by 20%.

Other studies have also found that processed meats increase your risk of colon cancer by 50%, bladder cancer by 59%, stomach cancer by 38%, and pancreatic cancer by 67%. Furthermore, bacon, hot dogs and other processed meats can increase your risk of type II diabetes by 50%, and decrease your lung function, increasing your risk for COPD (chronic obstructive pulmonary disease). Some animal products have an abundance of dioxins, yet another of the extremely toxic chemicals which has negative effects on the male reproductive system by lowering sperm count and the quality of sperm. Salicylates, naturally occurring chemicals in plants, many fruits, herbs, and vegetables that act as the natural immune hormone and preservative which protects the plants against diseases, insects, fungi, and harmful bacteria. A problem is that there are synthetically created salicylates interfering with Mother Nature. This man made form of salicylates can be found in many medicines, perfumes, and preservatives; they block the excretion of uric acid and can be responsible for some cases of gout. Phthalates, another highly toxic chemical to humans, also known as plasticizers, are the NUMBER ONE pollutant in the body. They are found in the plastic water bottles everybody is using because they believe them to be safe. Styrofoam cups leach these chemicals as well and are found everywhere in the wilderness and even in the stomachs in polar bears. They have been linked to diseases like osteoporosis and thyroid problems that some bears were found to have. More dangerous about these chemicals is that a pregnant mother's use of them will affect not only the unborn child's brain and glands, but its future fertility and maybe even cause cancer. Research today holds that phthalates cause obesity because they accumulate in the body and overwhelm its ability to detoxify them. In addition to the plastic water bottles and cups, phthalates can also be found in: auto exhausts, medications, flooring, construction materials, carpets, furniture, soda, infant formula, cosmetics, and nail polish as part of the infamous toxic trio. BHP or bisphenol A, a plasticizer, is another chemical found in plastic bottles with the recycle code of 3 or 7. These are also found in baby bottles and can leach out causing problems with the nervous and immune systems as well as disrupting the thyroid hormones. Furthermore, their use is linked to obesity, adult onset diabetes, ADD/ADHD, allergies, an increased risk for cancer and more. The fire retardant chemical is known as polybrominated diphenyl ethers or PHDE's; the use of these chemicals has been doubling every five years since 1972 and they have been found to contaminate all life around the globe, both human and animal. The foam in furniture and the pads under carpets are one source. This chemical also has been found to lower IQs.

There are also many toxic chemicals in household cleaners and personal hygiene products; toothpastes, soaps, shampoos, bath and shower gels, and products that lather and foam a lot contain a toxic chemical called sodium lauryl sulfate. This is probably the most dangerous ingredient used in skin and hair care products. A very highly corrosive and cheap detergent, it is used in the cleaning industry as a degreaser. Throughout the world it is used in clinical laboratories to irritate a test subject's skin so that researchers can then determine what will heal the skin. In other words, it is the most efficient skin irritant used for conducting experiments. It does this by drying the skin, striping off the lipid layer of the skin so the skin cannot regulate moisture. It can also cause hair loss when this skin protection is stripped, paving the way for skin rashes and infection.

Furthermore, this chemical will react with certain other chemicals in the skin care products to form nitrous amines or nitrates known to be carcinogens. Perhaps one of the most alarming characteristics of this chemical is the fact that it penetrates deep into certain tissues of the body and is stored there long-term. One study at the University of Georgia Medical College showed that it penetrated into the eyes, brain, heart and liver and when penetrated into children's eyes, retarded normal eye development. Furthermore, when penetrating adults' eyes, the study found it led to cataracts. Glycol ethers are another highly toxic solvent chemical found in cleaning products, cosmetics, brake fluids, and paint. Children exposed to this chemical- in the paint lining their bedroom walls, for example, were found to have higher rates of asthma and allergies.

In a recent article, from April of 2012, researchers examined nail polish in some hair salons and found toxins known as the "toxic trio": toluene, dibutyl phthalate, and formaldehyde. Exposure to large amounts of this trio is known to cause developmental problems and asthma. According to the California chemical regulators commission, who randomly sampled professional grade nail polishes that claimed to be free of this toxic trio, 121,000 licensed nail care technicians working in the salons-many of them young Asian American woman, are most at risk. I remember walking by a nail salon in a local mall last year and literally had to catch my breath because the vapors were so strong. Think about these workers exposed to these toxins day after day, year after year, FREE RADICAL DAMAGE at its finest.

The third component leading to free radical damage is heavy metal toxicity, occurring when certain metals in the environment get absorbed into our bodies. We can usually excrete them in ideal conditions so they do not build up in our system depending on exposure of course; however, unhealthy people and people with a certain genetic predisposition build up toxicity. The most common toxic heavy metals attacking the body are: mercury, aluminum, cadmium, arsenic and lead. Most anti-perspirants are loaded with aluminum, and the underarm is an easy portal of entry for these heavy metals to eventually accumulate. What is more dangerous, is the fact that some of these heavy metals can even have a negative synergistic effect. For example, one study showed a 100% mortality rate with test rats when they were exposed to small doses of both aluminum and mercury. Remember the HFCS (high fructose corn syrup) I just discussed earlier? There are many studies that detected mercury levels in HFCS. Crystalline fructose, a super potent form of fructose, the food and beverage industry is now using, may contain arsenic, lead, chloride, and other heavy metals.

Vaccinations, especially the DPT (Diphtheria, Polio and Tetanus vaccination) specifically, have aluminum and mercury as two of its ingredients which are causing heavy metal toxicity. Pandemrix, a flu shot vaccine, also has mercury as an ingredient. One Swedish study in June of 2012 reported that over 220 Swedes, most of them children, who received this swine flu shot, developed the sleeping disorder of narcolepsy. According to members of a support group formed for these victims, there are "a lot more undiagnosed cases." A father of one of the children affected said the disease is incurable, and that his son will have to go on heavy medication for the rest of his life. Another parent said of her son "it changed him; we've been robbed of our little fellow and our family life."

If we look at how the heavy metals get absorbed in our bodies, we have to look at the body's pH. Remember, the pH of the body is a measure of its mineral content and is supposed to be alkaline or basic; this means that our bodies should have an adequate mineral supply. When present, these minerals can compete with the heavy toxic metals in the environment getting into our bodies. Lead leaching from pipes into the water supply is a good example. Adequate levels of calcium, in the brush border cells that line our gut, prevent the absorption of heavy metals by competing with them. Thus, if there are not adequate minerals in our gut, there is nothing to compete with the heavy metals we ingest and consequently, they bio-accumulate.

A recent article posted on the Johnson Board by Dr. Walter Crooks, explains how the FASEB's (The Federation of American Societies for Experimental Biology) amalgam study revealed something shocking. The study found that there is a correlation between how many mercury fillings you have in your mouth and the amount of mercury in your brain because the hypothalamus and pituitary glands in your brain accumulate this heavy metal toxin. These two are the master glands that control all of your endocrine glands such as the thyroid, **parathyroid, which is the gland most susceptible to toxic heavy metals**, and the adrenals.

The article is titled: *Neurobehavioral effects from exposure to dental amalgam Hg: New distinctions between recent exposure and HG body burden*. Here is the URL if you would like to investigate more about this: http://www.fasebj.org/content/12/11/971.long.

Dr. Crooks, posted another article titled; "Oral galvanism and Electromagnetic Fields (EMF): factors along with mercury's high volatility and extreme toxicity in significant exposure levels and oral effects from amalgam fillings". (http://www.flcv.com/galv.htmll) He explains that mercury can leach out of the fillings ten times faster than normal if there is some type of galvanic reaction. This could be caused by having another type of metal in your mouth such as a crown, bridge, or retainer. For example, he states that electric current alone, known as galvanism, can cause brain fog and anxiety.

Remember, the Human body is alkaline by design and acidic by function. When we are sleeping our bodies try to heal and return to an alkaline pH by morning. As we go through the day, many of us eat the S.A.D. and are exposed to all the aforementioned chemicals and toxicities. As the day progresses our pH becomes more acidic unless it has a reserve of minerals to buffer the blood; without these minerals the body will take calcium out of the bones to buffer the blood in order to raise the pH. This is known as micro-crystalline hydroxyapatite and can potentially lead to osteoporosis. Also, without the necessary minerals the thyroid hormone, T3, cannot get into the cells. Hence the importance of the thyroid comes up again. Because the thyroid is the spark plug for energy production, every cell has thyroid receptors; moreover it helps with childhood growth, regulates body temperature, and has a huge influence on brain chemistry, mainly moods and emotion. We now can add mineral deficiency causing pH imbalance, along with the white flour I discussed earlier as a probable contributor to the possibly 30 million undiagnosed thyroid problems. If this is not bad enough we cannot ignore the parathyroid, a small gland that surrounds the thyroid. Its main job is to maintain the body's calcium level by buffering the blood making more alkaline when it becomes to acidic. It is supposed to buffer the blood or make the blood more alkaline when the body becomes too acidic. With all of the acidic people out there guess what? Their Parathyroid is not functioning. Why, you ask? The reason is that it needs minerals and VIT D, which I will talk about very soon. Remember, however, you have to be acidic before this can happen; having a pH in the acidic range, for a long period of time makes it easy for your health to take a downward spiral. Bacteria and viruses love an acidic environment; cancer, for example, thrives in an acidic environment.

Again let me summarize. Low or acidic pH is caused by mineral deficiency mostly the result of an improper S.A.D. For heavy metals to bio-accumulate when anyone is exposed to them, either environmentally, as pollution, or from food and water sources, he must be ACIDIC. This heavy metal toxicity may then lead to chronic illness. PH is a logarithmic scale; this simply means that for each 10th of a point that your pH drops, there is a 10 fold shift in effect. Americans have become more acidic over the past decade, dropping the average pH range by 5 tenths of a point.

I will briefly discuss excitotoxins, a fancy word for neurotransmitters which can cause a cell to die when their actions are prolonged. A neurotransmitter is a chemical released from a nerve cell which is a messenger of nerve information from one cell to another. Some examples of excitotoxins are glutamate, in monosodium glutamate or MSG from dining out, and aspartate or aspartame, aka NutraSweet. A poster on naturalnews.com stated "aspartame is linked to leukemia and lymphoma," and added that this is related to a new landmark study on humans. The researchers found that drinking one can of 12 ounce diet soda per day increased their rate of developing Leukemia by 42%, multiple myeloma, a serious cancer, by 102%, and non-Hodgkin's lymphoma by 31%. These finding were all in comparison with participants who drank NO diet soda. In the United States diet soda is the largest source of aspartame; Americans consume about 5,250 tons of aspartame per year, of which 85% or 4,500 tons is from drinking diet sodas. Rats subjected to aspartame over their whole lives from fetal development also showed increased lymphoma and leukemia rates as well as an increased breast cancer rate. For those of you, who think you might as well just drink the sugar filled soda, don't be so hasty. The human study also showed that men who drank one or more sugar sweetened soda daily had a 66% increase in non-Hodgkin's lymphoma. This is almost double the risk of the diet soda. I am sure the sugar source from the sweetened non-diet soda was HFCS and not natural cane sugar.

Speaking of sweeteners let me tell you about sucralose, also known as Splenda, introduced in late 1999 and best known for its marketing ploy, "made from sugar so it tastes like sugar." From 2000-2004 the number of households using it jumped from 3 to 20%. The sales of splenda were $177 million versus the $62 million spent on equal which is aspartame based and $52 million on Sweet 'N Low which is saccharine based. The advertising company, McNeil Nutritionals, wanted to really emphasize how rigorous the safety studies were on Splenda and they boasted of over 100 clinical trials. What they do not state is that most of them were done on animals. There have only been six human trials on Splenda to date. Before FDA approval there were only two or so studies involving a few dozen people that lasted only 4 days. After FDA approval, a human toxicity study was conducted for only three months, which is the longest clinical study on Splenda to date. They have no study information on the effects of Splenda on children or pregnant woman.

Sucralose starts out as a sugar molecule but then becomes a highly processed synthetic chemical in the factory. I need to be a little technical here to make a point; bear with me. Three chlorine molecules are added to the sugar molecule which is a disaccharide of glucose and fructose. At the factory to make sucralose, they alter the chemical composition of sugar so much that it is converted to fructo-galactose molecule in a five step chemical process. Like the GMO (genetically modified) wheat, corn and salmon, your body does not recognize this type of sugar molecule and, therefore, it cannot properly break it down in your system. Thus the marketing claim by McNeil Nutritionals about its not having any calories is justified in their minds because of this "unique biochemical make-up." The zero calories only come into play because your body cannot use it. This brings me to the next point of how much is left in your body, and what are the effects of ingesting it?

If we look at some of the animal studies we see that 15% of sucralose is stored and absorbed in the digestive tract. There was a human study with 8 participants. Even after three days, none of the eight excreted any of the sucralose. Their bodies had to be absorbing it right? If you have a healthy digestive tract you are more prone to metabolize and break down the sucralose. What does this mean to you the consumer who has been consuming this advertised safe chemical for years with reckless abandonment? I have been out to eat with people over the years who bought into this seductive advertising. I can remember people just dumping packet after packet of this junk into their iced tea saying, "no calories just great taste." I remember saying to myself, "If they need their drink to be that sweet in the first place, then they have problems." Remember folks, 15% of it stays with you. Because of its chemical altering, Splenda is really more like the pesticide DDT than it is like sugar. And the storage of 15% of it in your fat cells for years and years cannot be a good thing. Nobody really knows what its long-term effects are.

In one of the human studies that lasted a month, ingesting 500 mg/kg of sucralose caused lesions in the liver and kidneys. Keep in mind, however, that this is about 34 grams for average 150 pound adult or 680 packets of Splenda. But to be practical we are really talking about the habitual use of the product. This is not a onetime food additive. One of the other human studies, I referenced at least five out of the six so far, points to changes in the intestinal flora and the altering of pH in human waste. This occurred at a 1.1- 11 mg/kg dose. This is very doable for the same 150 pound adult or about 1.5 packets of splenda/sucralose per day.

Another excitotoxin is homocysteine which can be generated in response to a toxic or nutritionally deficient diet of B6, B12, folic acid, and magnesium. These excitotoxins can cause cell death by initiating a mutation or alteration of a gene known as P53. This "guardian angel gene" as it is called, causes cell apoptosis, or cell death by suicide. In particular, the microglial cell which is an immature central nervous system cell wreaks havoc on the body when these excitotoxins are present causing massive amounts of inflammation and destruction of tissues which leads to many of the degenerative diseases such as Alzheimer's. When aluminum is bound to the excitotoxins glutamate (MSG) or aspartame (aka E Coli poop), its entry into your brain is significantly elevated. Once in the brain, aluminum increased iron induced free radical activity.

This is an appropriate time to bring up the subject of the United States' philosophy versus Europe's on food and environmental safety. I watched many You-tube videos devoted to this very subject that stressed its importance in contributing to the declining health of this country. There are several foods and chemicals that are banned in Europe and allowed in the United States. Let's look at ten examples.

1. **Most genetically modified foods** (high fructose corn syrup – a genetically modified food – is banned in Europe).

2. **All antibiotics and related drugs fed to livestock** for growth promotion purposes (like Bovine Growth Hormone).

3. **22 pesticides used on crops** (banned by EU (European Union)) – not approved by all countries yet.

4. **Chickens washed in chlorine**. All chickens exported from the United States are washed in chlorine and, therefore, not allowed in Europe.

5. **Different standard for approving food contact products** with chemicals in them (i.e. plastic bottles for water, milk etc.) – EU requires that the manufacturer PROVES safety or it will be banned. Biphenyl A (BPA) in baby bottles is banned.

6. **Synthetic food colors** i.e. Red 40, Yellow 5, Yellow 6, Blue 1, Blue 2, Green 3, Orange B, and Red 3 (used heavily in candy, breakfast cereals and even yoghurt).

7. **Irradiation to kill dangerous organisms** in beef, pork, chicken, lamb, herbs, spices, flour and fruit and vegetables. The EU only permits it on dried spices, herbs and vegetable based seasonings.

8. **Bleached flour** – (used in all white bread and some wheat bread.)

9. **Partially hydrogenated oil** - most European countries completely ban it or severely restrict it.

10. **Many chemicals such as aspartame and saccharine / preservatives like titanium dioxide** used as sugar substitutes and to make food white, bright and in other products like toothpaste.

I have heard on more than one occasion that someone gluten intolerant went to Europe for a trip and slipped up by eating gluten, only to suffer no ill effects. Wine has the same effect. In America most wine has sulfates added to act as a preservative. These sulfates are naturally occurring anyway as the yeast ferments in grape skins. They are a natural byproduct of this process to prevent bacteria growth and spoilage. Naturally they occur at about 10 parts per million and do not need to even be on the label. When you add them, however, they cause problems to some people, like asthmatics, for example. Others get bad headaches after drinking wine with added sulfates.

The common philosophy of the United States on this subject seems to be that a food or chemical is innocent or harmless until proven guilty or harmful. European philosophy on the same matter has it opposite; a product is considered harmful or guilty until proven harmless or innocent.

CHAPTER SIX

Sick at the Cellular Level:
Depleted Methyl Groups

We have discussed in detail the free radical activity and excitotoxins components of why so many of us are unhealthy. I will describe how our organs, particularly the liver and gallbladder are affected all the way down to the DNA level of the cell.

The gallbladder's function is to store and concentrate bile, which is made in the liver, and then to release it into the small intestine to further digest food, especially fats. I am SHOCKED to find out many of my patients had their gallbladder's removed because of stones and were never told about the importance of supplementation.

This Bile has two major functions in the body. It breaks down the fat you ingest so your body can utilize them. Without adequate amounts of bile, your body cannot properly break down and absorb fat soluble vitamins. This means you will be deficient in the fat-soluble vitamins A, D, E, and K - not to mention essential fatty acids. If this affects you, some symptoms could be dry skin, such as peeling on the soles of your feet, and constipation.

Bile is also a very powerful antioxidant against FREE RADICALS. I hope you see how all of this ties together. This antioxidant, bile, helps to remove toxins from the liver. Toxins could be bacteria, viruses, drugs, and any foreign substances your body does not want. The toxins then travel with the bile through the bile duct of the liver to the gallbladder or directly to the small intestine. Here it will join the waste matter to be excreted through the colon with the feces. For those who have gallbladder problems, one must look at the liver and colon. Constipation is a common sign that gallbladder stress is present. It is also caused by not drinking enough water. If you are over forty, the S.A.D. has definitely had an impact on your normal gallbladder function. The nutrient that keeps the bile salts in suspension preventing stagnation and a clog in the gallbladder, which then can lead to stones, is vitamin B6. This vitamin is depleted by stress, estrogen in birth control pills, etc. **Some contend that women who were EVER on the birth control pill may have depleted their B6 vitamin stores so that they need to take a supplement of B6 for life, or else they will not be able to absorb fats.** Many of you reading this take Vitamin D and essential fatty acid supplements, however, due to the above statement are not absorbing it in sufficient amount, if at all. **You must look at the gallbladder and liver.**

This brings us to the liver. Here are some of its normal functions: bile production and excretion, excretion of bilirubin, cholesterol, hormones, drugs, metabolism of proteins, fats, and carbohydrates, enzyme activation, storage of glycogen, vitamins, and minerals, synthesis of plasma proteins, such as albumin, and clotting factors. Finally, it detoxifies and purifies the blood. One can see why this organ is so important to your body's overall health.

I have discussed how these two organs are affected; let's take it one step further and look at the gene level. I know this is a little confusing but the easier explanation is coming up next. Dr. Johnson does an excellent job explaining how diseases begin at the cell level. He considers how we develop a chronic disease by asking: "Did you ever wonder why all of a sudden someone comes down with a chronic disease or even cancer? It was not from a spell or curse. It did not just fall from the sky and land on their head. No, they had a bad gene expressed instead of suppressed like a healthy body maintains. This is from depleted methyl groups". For any chemistry buffs out there reading this, a methyl (CH3) is part of an acetyl group (COCH3). How do we express a bad gene? Well, the answer is methyl groups or in this cases the lack of them. **How do we deplete methyl groups? By consuming the S.A.D., which is high in WHITE FLOUR, WHITE SALT, AND WHITE SUGAR - AKA "WHITE DEATH", TRANS FATTY ACIDS, HYDROGENATED OILS, PESTICIDES, CAFFEINE LAIDEN DRINKS, PRODUCE LOADED WITH PESTICIDES AND HERBACIDES, HIGH FRUCTOSE CORN SYRUP, GENETICALLY MODIFIED FOODS, AND - last but not least - STRESS!!**

What creates methyl groups? Hydrochloric acid (HCL) or stomach acid does, and you need the proper amount of it to create methyl groups. The problem is we produce less HCL as we age. And the poor diet and stress that I have been harping on this whole chapter also deplete it. You also need these methyl groups for cell replication at the level of the DNA. Remember that I explained that this same cellular DNA is also 10 times more vulnerable to free radical damage. When you have enough methyl groups or methylation you have good genes like tumor suppressor genes turned "on" and bad genes like onco genes turned "off." Without sufficient methyl groups you have the opposite, where the oncogenes, or bad genes, turned "on" and the tumor suppressing genes or good genes turned "off".

These methyl groups are also needed for phase two liver detoxification, protein methylation, and neurotransmitter synthesis. You remember neurotransmitters; I talked about dopamine, a neurotransmitter that affects your movement and coordination.

To summarize, someone will succumb to a chronic disease once his methyl groups are depleted. He will then come in contact with a toxin of some sort. It could even be electromagnetic exposure like a cell phone tower or constant cell phone use. He could have had some dental work, maybe a death in the family or are going through a divorce. In other words he had a period of HIGH STRESS and then BOOM... the bad gene is expressed. This can mean that a person may develop a neurodegenerative disorder like MS, an autoimmune disorder like rheumatoid arthritis, or even cancer. Remember, the initial cause of these chronic diseases is depleted methyl groups. This sets the stage or allows the diseases to occur.

I was going to end this topic right here but I just recently read an article on pathogenic mycoplasma that contends that this toxin is the primary culprit for many of the chronic diseases we suffer from. I will briefly discuss this topic with you so that you can decide whether you would like to investigate further.

Most mycoplasma is harmless and there are over 200 species. Only about 4 or 5 are pathogenic or cause disease. During 1942 and the present time, biological warfare research has resulted in more deadly infectious forms of mycoplasma. The one I am talking about is Mycoplasma Fermentans. It comes from the nucleus of the Brucella bacterium which is not really a bacterium or a virus but a mutant form of the Brucella bacterium combined with a virus. The mycoplasma is then taken out of it. This was then actually reduced to a crystalline form and then it was tested on an unsuspecting North America. Dr. Mark Hilleman, chief virologist for Merck, stated that this disease agent is carried by EVERYONE IN NORTH AMERICA AND POSSIBLY MOST PEOPLE THROUGHOUT THE WORLD.

Could this be another cause for all of the increase in chronic neurodegenerative diseases since WWII? Dr. Shyh-Ching Lo, senior researcher at The Armed Forces Institute of Pathology, and one of America's top mycoplasma researchers, feels that this disease agent causes many illnesses including AIDS, cancer, chronic fatigue syndrome, Chrohn's, colitis, Type I diabetes, multiple sclerosis, rheumatoid arthritis, Parkinson's, and Alzheimer's. Dr. Charles Engel, who is with the National Institutes of Health in Maryland, said at a November 2000 meeting, "I am now of the view that the probable cause of chronic fatigue syndrome and fibromyalgia is the mycoplasma…"

This mycoplasma agent is not really known by the medical profession because it was developed by the US military in biological warfare experimentation and it was not made public. It was actually patented by the US military and Dr. Shyh-Ching Lo. In the 1940's all of the countries at war were experimenting with biological weapons. The US, Canada, and Britain entered into an agreement whereby they would develop one biological weapon that would kill and one that was disabling. They primarily focused on the Brucella bacterium and began to weaponize it. These diseases were around for thousands of years, but now they were made more contagious and more effective.

This article continues to explain that many senators and members of congress had no idea that this was going on. When it was brought to their attention, the US Senate Committee on Government Reform searched the archives for certain documents and could not find them. They are presently trying to stop this type of biological research.

With the crystalline form, the disease agent can be stored, transported, and deployed without deteriorating. It could be delivered by insects, aerosol, or the food chain. The factor that is working in the Brucella is the mycoplasma. This disease agent, Brucella, doesn't kill people, it disables them. In 1969, researchers found that if the mycoplasma had certain strength - 10 to the 10th power - it would develop AIDS and the person would die quickly because it could bypass the body's natural defenses. However, if the strength of mycoplasma was 10 to 8th power, chronic fatigue or fibromyalgia would develop in the person. If it was 10 to 7th power then the person would simply seem to be wasting away and not very interested in life. That does sound like many of the chronic disease patients today.

The disease Brucellosis disappeared once we started pasteurizing milk, which was the carrier. If you never drank cow's milk you may not have been exposed. It is eerie to think, however, that one salt shaker full of this pure disease agent in crystalline form could sicken the entire population of Canada. It is very deadly, not in terms of killing but because it is so disabling.

In a patient's blood, mycoplasma will only crystallize at a pH of 8.1. Blood has a pH of 7.4 so doctors do not even look for it. So how do you know if this is affecting you? There is a test called "The Polymerase Chain Reaction Test". The mycoplasma organism is very small; in fact it is so minute that normal blood and tissue tests will not reveal its presence as the source of the disease. Until thirty years ago when this test was developed, the mycoplasma could not even be detected. Here, damaged particles in your blood are removed and subjected to a polymerase chain reaction. This causes the DNA in the particles to break down. These particles are then placed in a nutrient, which causes the DNA to grow back to its original form. If enough of the substance is produced, the form can be recognized. It can then be determined whether Brucella or another kind of agent is behind that particular mycoplasma.

If anybody in your family has fibromyalgia, multiple sclerosis, or Alzheimer's, you can send a blood sample to Dr. Les Simpson in New Zealand for testing. Blood cells normally have a doughnut shape which can be compressed and squeezed through capillaries. The blood cells in a mycoplasma infected person swell up and cannot be compressed because they lose their flexibility. Guess what gives the blood cells their flexibility? Cholesterol does. Yes, that is right. It is good to talk about cholesterol in a positive light. The mycoplasma feeds on the cholesterol in the red blood cells so they cannot go through blood vessels. The person then feels the aches and pains of the damage it causes to the brain, heart, stomach, feet, and the whole body because blood and oxygen are cut off. Do these not sound like fibromyalgia and chronic fatigue syndrome symptoms?

To diagnose chronic fatigue syndrome and fibromyalgia doctors have patients wear a Holter ECG for 24 hours. This tests shows that 100% of people with chronic fatigue syndrome and fibromyalgia have an irregular heartbeat. One of the waves with the heartbeat, the "T" wave, will flatten or actually invert. This means blood is not being squeezed through the big blood vessel, called the aorta, and sent through the body.

Lastly, another test to diagnose the disease is the Blood Volume Test. Every human requires a certain amount of blood per pound of body weight. Chronic fatigue, fibromyalgia, multiple sclerosis, and other such illness patients do not have the normal blood volume their body needs to function properly. Doctors are not usually aware of this. This test uses 5cc of the patients' blood and puts a tracer on it. After the blood is put back into the body a technician looks for the tracer. The thicker the blood and the lower blood volume, the more tracers you will find.

If it is carried by all of us, some are genetically predisposed to get really sick and others will not even be affected by mycoplasma. Keep in mind that if you are not genetically predisposed yet eat the S.A.D. diet and/or are exposed to many toxic chemicals and heavy metals, you are opening up the door to more damage. If you do everything right and still succumb to this then you have to find a way to stop the mycoplasma growth long enough for your immune system to take over and defeat it.

CHAPTER SEVEN

It's Stress!

Even the AMA (American Medical Association) agrees that 85% of all disease is due to some form of STRESS. When I went over all of the causes of why we are so sick, in reality I was talking about the things that are causing the most "stress" to our bodies. They could be chemical, physical, and emotional. Obviously, the things related to diet, toxic chemicals, and drugs are chemical stressors. These can also cause physical stress. Look at someone having a pollen reaction that is sneezing like crazy with a runny nose and swollen nasal membranes. So many times a chemical stressor causes a physical stress to the body that can also affect the emotions. A person with pollen allergies is very stressed and anxious when outside and the grass is being mowed. During the pollen season, until the first frost, is an anxious time for these people. I want you to get the point that the negative effects on both the body and mind are acting as stressors.

A person sweating out his utility bill this month, an expectant mother worrying about the health of her baby, and a soldier undergoing basic training all have one thing in common-**STRESS**. There is a general adaption period to stress. First we have alarm, where there is a reaction. A great example is an anaphylactic response where someone's throat closes when stung by a bee. Next we have the resistance stage where we fight the stressor. The nervous and endocrine systems play the largest part in this stage by trying to maintain what is known as homeostasis or balance in the body. Finally, we have the exhaustion stage where we can no longer fight. This is where disease comes in. Due to all the stressors we are under, our bodies are overcome, our immune system becomes compromised, and we succumb to a less than optimal state or a disease - a state of being away from health.

One purpose of this book then is to try to steer you away from unnecessary stressors. Yes we are all exposed to stress on a daily basis. Some stress is healthy; for example if we did not have to deal with gravity our muscles would atrophy and shrivel up. So we need exercise and resistance training to build up and maintain our bodies. This brings to mind the line from Kelly Clarkson's recent hit, "What doesn't kill you makes you stronger." This adaption to stress is amazing. The epitome of stress adaption would be that of a professional bodybuilder where the muscles grew beyond what Mother Nature intended. Thus building muscle is a stress adaption response to a physical stressor.

When discussing why so many of us are so unhealthy we must not forgo something called the epigenetic connection. There is an article written by Dr. Theresa Dale which delves into how our emotions influence our DNA. With all of the depression out there and stress with the economy, people in this country are just trying to stay afloat, let alone get ahead. This all leaves many of us on an emotional roller coaster. Here is something very interesting that we all must keep in mind when it comes to being sick or healthy. Traditional science has held that our genes are fixed and nothing can change genetic determination. Epigenetics is all based on a three thousand year old Chinese philosophy of the five elements and the circadian rhythm which is your sleep cycle. It refers to the relationship between emotions and disease. Each element is related to an organ in the body and a certain emotion and is used in Chinese medicine to diagnose disharmony and disease. Each emotion has a certain electromagnetic energy pattern. Since acupuncture meridians are bioactive energy pathways corresponding to various organs and glands, and each organ stores specific emotions, one can easily see the relationship between disease and thoughts. When you harbor negative thoughts and they get into your subconscious mind, the information gets transmitted into all of your cells. Research today has also found that genetics are controlled by the perception of our environment - not genes. Genes do not just control who you are or your biological expression; they also adapt to your beliefs and identities. Genes cannot turn themselves on or off. The organism changes to adapt to the environment. Dr. Dale explains a process that must occur for the structure of the gene to be altered. This should be a familiar term to you by now. It is methylation of a cell. Again, this turns on good genes and turn off bad genes. If methylation of DNA is prevented or limited, embryos will not develop and life just stops. This is important information we are talking about here. The methylation of DNA was the first epigenetic change to be observed in cancer cells. I discussed this in the excitotoxins section. The rock iron and decreased stomach acid all equal small amounts of B vitamins which means decrease methylation and increased aging and cancer. Additionally, there are arsenic and cadmium I talked about in the toxic heavy metal section which also impair DNA methylation.

I want you to come away with the thought that not only does the bad nutrition and toxic chemicals alter our DNA, but ANYTHING causing increased stress levels makes this happen easier. Dr. Dale says, "Stress is that uncomfortable gap between how you would like your life to be and how it actually is."

When dealing with the reasons we are so sick, for example- where the adaption period cannot fully occur, we can come down with a chronic disease. This is when the "bad genes" are being expressed and the "good genes" are being turned off. A look at the physiology of what happens to the body when we are under a lot of stress will be helpful.

When dealing with any type of stress we must mention the Adrenal glands. These tiny glands, which sit on top of the kidneys, act like the battery in your car, and respond to ANY STRESSOR, no matter what it may be. This is like the guy who shoots first and asks questions later.

The adrenal glands want you to be prepared and able to handle any situation thrown at them. In this way the human body is an incredible machine with all systems working synergistically. The adrenal glands, along with the thyroid gland, have the greatest blood supply per ounce of tissue having up to 60 arterioles which are small blood vessels supplying the tissue with oxygen rich blood. This stress can be real or perceived. The body will respond the same. The stress can also be from inside the body or outside the body; the body does not know the difference. Yes, you read it right. The adrenal glands will respond to a perceived fear or stressor in the same way it would if the stressor was real. And brief or long-term stress both weakens the capability of your adrenal glands to deal with stressors. When your body is presented with a stressor and is in the alarm state, it tries to gather all of its resources to respond. Its first response is epinephrine or adrenaline; this is the fight or flight hormone that is supposed to get you out of a jam. You may or may not have heard of feats of super human strength, as the case of a mother who lifted a car off her son when it fell on him. This hormone is responsible for that response. Along with this hormone, however, another one called cortisol is also released and continues to be released until the perceived threat is gone, and the brain tells the adrenal glands to stop secreting it. So the brief stress hormone released is the adrenaline and the long-term stress hormone secreted is cortisol. The problem is that when the stressors never stop, the cortisol keeps coming. The body is not designed for this, therefore; other functions will suffer and be impaired. The other systems affected by the actions of cortisol are: cardiovascular system, central nervous system, immune system, brain, bone health, thyroid, and protein, carbohydrate, and fat metabolism. One of the major effects on the body by constant release of cortisol from stress is catabolism or the breaking down of tissue, the opposite of anabolism, or the building up of tissue as in gaining muscle. Collagen is reduced by a factor of ten with increased cortisol. Collagen is what holds tissue together including the skin. **This**

is why excess exposure to stress makes people look older. The consequences of stress are all encompassing. I want you to see how stressors can be traced back from all disease processes. There is weakness, unexplained hair loss, nervousness, lowered body temperature, depression, irritability, hypoglycemia, difficulty gaining weight, inability to concentrate, excessive hunger, tendency toward inflammation, poor memory/confusion, digestive dysfunction, feelings of frustration, overall feeling of ill-health, osteoporosis, auto-immune disease, heart palpitations, dizziness upon standing, lowered resistance to infections, high blood pressure, insomnia, sweet/salt cravings, and headaches.

Keep in mind that after a long period of cortisol elevation from chronic stressors, your system will crash, and you will have lower cortisol levels. The symptoms are pretty much the same with this crash, there is going to be a low blood pressure with extreme fatigue and weight gain tendencies. When your cortisol crashes after it has been high for so long, you are in what is called "adrenal fatigue." These symptoms are indicative of those people being diagnosed with chronic fatigue syndrome and "fibromyalgia" – the mystery diagnosis that really means, "I do not know what is wrong with you." Mostly what patients complain about is that their sleep cycle is "all screwed up." Normally, your circadian rhythm has your cortisol highest in the morning to wake you up and then it gradually declines to its lowest level at night so you can fall asleep and stay asleep. Sleeping pills such as Ambien do not address the cause or try to normalize your cortisol levels with the normal sleep pattern. Instead their mechanism is to make the cell receptors that let the neurotransmitter GABA in, up to 7 to 10 times more sensitive. One of GABA's functions is to aid the body in sleep. How tired is one going to get if 7-10 times the amount of GABA are instantly allowed into your cells? The result is almost a trance. This pill is quickly overtaking illegal sedatives in becoming the most popular date rape drug due to its hypnotic tendencies. Let's just say after only two weeks, it can be highly addictive and cause a list of serious side effects. I will have some answers to why many people cannot sleep later. **I hope you now see how harmful stressors are the problem. You need to avoid the harmful stressors in order to be healthier.**

CHAPTER EIGHT

The Medical Profession's Answers to Your Health

With the health of this country going downhill fast, statistics project that this latest generation is the first ever that may outlive their parents because of, "poor health". We spend around a whopping $900 billion of our national budget on healthcare yet we rank about 30th in the world in infant mortality.

Look at these shocking statistics: With all of this gun debate sparked due to the recent tragedies at shopping malls and elementary schools, we cannot lose sight of the bigger picture of controllable deaths in this country. Look at some statistics from 2011 from "Natural News." The number of deaths in this country from guns breaks down as follows: Homicide- 11,101, Suicide-19,766, Unintentional shooting- 851, and undetermined intent- 222 for a total of **31,940** deaths in this country. When we look at the number deaths from the United States Medical system it breaks down as follows: Adverse drug reactions- 106,000, Outpatients- 199,000, Medical errors- 98,000, other medical related- 380,936 for a grand total of **783,936. This is the total number of iatrogenic (caused by the physician) deaths.** The American medical system is the leading cause of death and injury in the United States. And keep in mind that there are 2 million adverse drug reactions with serious side effects aside from the 106,000 deaths each year. Additionally, here are a couple more mind blowing facts about the medical system. There are 7.5 million unnecessary surgical procedures done each year. And the number of people exposed to unnecessary hospitalization is 8.9 million annually. An article on Yahoo recently stated that hospitals are tripling their profits from surgical mishaps. This is from a study in JAMA (Journal of the American Medical Association), which analyzed 34,256 inpatient surgical procedures performed in 2010 at 12 hospitals run by Texas Health Resources, a large non-profit hospital system. The average boost in profits was $30,500 per patient from a PREVENTABLE surgical complication. The reason is that insurance plans paid for the extra stay and care involved. The study reveals how hospitals are rewarded for surgical mistakes; the prize for hospitals striving to improve patient safety and reduce surgical errors is less money. The JAMA editorial written with the article states, that this practice should be the "impetus for payment reform."

Furthermore, prescription drugs kill almost 300 people per day, 365 days per year. For gun massacres to be even close to these numbers there would have to be a mass shooting every hour of every day, 365 days per year. This is something to keep in perspective. If a jet crashed every day 365 days per year in this country, do you think the American public would stand for it?

This brings me to my next point. As I write this I feel a little trepidation that I should look over my shoulder... Big Pharma has SO MUCH MONEY. According to an article by Dr. Christopher Kent, "Our Drug Problem: Fighting the Wrong Enemy", recreational drugs such as cocaine and heroin kill anywhere between 10,000 and 15,000 per year. This is a serious health problem but only pales in comparison to the prescription drug deaths numbers I alluded to above. How do the drug companies lure us in, so to speak? There is another article written by Dr. J.C Smith, which is titled "Medical Payola". This refers to how, just like the old radio days when the disc jockeys were bribed to play certain records, Big Pharma was found guilty in a Senate investigation in a multi-million dollar bribery scheme where they paid medical doctors millions to push their brand name drugs. Eighty four percent of medical doctors from 2004 - 2009 admitted to a financial relationship with a drug company. From 2009 to mid-2011, there was $769 million paid to medical doctors. One cannot disagree, however, that any research funded by a drug company is suspect. For instance, there are situations where the drug companies fly researchers around first class, and later the researcher will deliver a company slide show or speech. There are the ghostwriters in the drug industry that pays an honorarium to put their names on articles and submit them to a peer review journal. Lastly, there are drug companies who hire researchers as consultants to give them advice. In fact, 28% of medical doctors polled admitted that they received "honorariums" of up to $6000 per day from a drug company to serve on an advisory board or as a consultant. In 2010, drug companies spent a whopping $220 million on speaking fees to doctors who pushed their drug. Why do the drug companies do this? Former editor and chief of The New England Journal of Medicine, Marcia Angell, said it is because those researchers, who give speeches, write journal articles and textbooks are worth 100,000 salesmen. Drug companies make money. How much money? Let's just say the between 1995 and 2010 profits rose by $200 billion.

The AMA had been linked to corruption long before big pharma was in the picture. Many people do not realize, I did not, that in 1930 the AMA accepted advertisements from the tobacco industry. It was under the leadership of a Morris Fishbein MD, executive director, and also senior editor of the Journal of the American Medical Association. This made the AMA the most powerful lobby in the world. They wanted to snuff out any competition, including chiropractic, but were unsuccessful thank goodness. So, in the 1940s you had the journal with millions of dollars of tobacco advertising. I remember a patient who spent over a year in the hospital with 56 surgeries or so. He used to tell me that all of the doctors and nurses would gather in his room and smoke. This was in the 1970s. If your doctor was smoking it must be good for you, right? In 1986 with all of the mounting evidence over the harmful effects of tobacco and cigarette smoke, public pressure forced the tobacco-AMA marriage to divorce. This is where big pharma comes in. When the tobacco company was out, Big Pharma was in to replace the lost income. Nowhere more than in Congress, does money talk. Yet, as I have stated, we spend the most on healthcare but have a terrible record on the health of our population. Dr. Smith brings up a great point in his medical payola article when he says that nobody from the AMA, big pharma, big hospitals, or big insurance ever was called on Capitol Hill to testify as to why this is true. Let's look at what big pharma, The Hospital Association, BC/BS, and the AMA spent on lobbying from 1998-2008. Big pharma spent $154,533,400, the American Hospital Association $172,940,431, Blue Cross/Blue Shield $120,491,385, and the American Medical Association $208,472,500. This information can be obtained from Opensecrets.org. If we add that up it comes to $656,437,716. Divide this sum by 535 members of congress and you get $1,226,986 for each member.

This article gives some examples of surgical costs. By the way, most of you know that back surgery is about 50% successful- sort of like the marriage/divorce rate. It is like rolling the dice. According to an author of The Backletter, a newsletter from the Department of Orthopedic Surgery at Georgetown Medical Center in Washington D.C., "Spinal treatment is the poster child for inefficient spinal care". Dr. Gordon Waddell, an orthopedist and author, wrote "Low Back pain has been a 20th century health care disaster... back surgery has been accused of leaving more tragic human wreckage in its wake than any other operation in history." Another author in the Backletter made reference to the increasing frustration with the medical approach to low back pain: "The world of spinal medicine unfortunately is producing patients with failed back surgery syndrome at an alarming rate...there is little evidence that the patient outcomes have improved." I do not even know how to respond to those two statements, except maybe to see justification for what I have been preaching to patients for the past twenty-five years. Just like Big Pharma, the surgical instrument and hardware companies do their own share of medical payola. The Senate Finance Committee found that the medical device companies were corrupting surgeons, and medical journals were publishing articles that were edited by medical researchers on the take.

Listen to how blatant this is. In 2009, Medtronic, the biggest maker of spinal implants accounted for half of the worldwide income of $7 billion. For spinal fusions they make pedicle screws which sell for $2,000 - $3,000 A PIECE? One surgeon was quoted as saying, "You can easily put $30,000 of hardware in a person during a fusion." Medtronic also edited medical journal articles written by physicians who downplayed the risks of "infuse"- the company's beset selling bone graft. They would use this powerful biological agent which is a bone growth stimulant instead of the patient's own bone. This infuse would sell for around $5,000 per pack. When the Senate Finance Committee investigated Medtronic, they found that the world's largest medical device maker did not disclose its role in shaping 13 key studies involving the use of infuse which made Medtronic an $800 million a year profit. One clinical trial of infuse was halted because 70% of the participants experienced excessive boney growth in the spinal canals. This will cause spinal stenosis leading to more surgery. Other side effects of infuse were found to be: male sterility, infection, and increased back and leg pain. Hmm, just like the commercials where the side effects include the same symptoms as the drug is trying to suppress. Remember the 50% success rate? Fusions really bring down the success rate and cost Medicare $343 million in 1997 and $2.24 billion in 2008 - a 400% increase. In spite of the success/fail rate do you think there may be a slight financial incentive to do fusions? Lastly, you are not going to believe what the medical device companies will pay these surgeons for surgeries. One surgeon from Memphis's Methodist University Hospital was paid royalties from Medtronic since 1996. He received $26 million from

2001 - 2006. On Medtronic's own website they describe how in the first two quarters of 2011 they paid him royalties of $13 million.

Just remember the theme here, from the tobacco and pharmaceuticals companies, to surgical corruption. We have bias, bribery and greed. Due to the great advertising and marketing of the medical professionals and medical media, however, most people do not know this history. Yes there have been and will be many more future lawsuits but until the public wakes up, the medical profession will continue to take advantage of them.

 In this country about 2/3 of whites and 3/4 of Hispanics and blacks are considered overweight with 1/3 of whites and Hispanics, and 1/5 of blacks being considered obese - where one's overall body fat is 30% or greater. For the first time in history, we are seeing kids with obesity and all of the problems that go with it such as high blood pressure, high cholesterol, and what used to be adult onset type II diabetes.

I must mention the inactivity factor of today's generation. Remember the family with the overweight kids I wrote about in the introduction who gave me the idea to write this book? These kids were riding their bikes on that day at least. For the most part, kids today would rather play video games than do something physical. I can honestly say, I never got into the Xbox thing but my daughters still had excuses not to play outside much when they were little. I remember one year when it was snowing out and they said they wanted to sleigh ride at the school across the street. After five minutes, they said, "It is too cold out here," and came in. I also remember one summer day when they wanted to play outside on the custom-made swing play set I built for them. The play session also lasted for about fifteen minutes. They came in stomping their foot announcing that it is "Just too hot outside." They were probably in the ten to twelve age ranges at the time. I thought how things changed since I was a kid. Now as I am writing this, about ten years later, I see this lack of physical activity on the rise even more. Kids spend something like FIVE HOURS A DAY on some form of electronic media. It would be amazing what they could accomplish in a day if they used the energy they expend with technology on something useful like exercise and reading.

Furthermore, there's the "pill for every ill" philosophy instilled in our kids at an early age. We teach them to think of drugs whenever there is pain. I have a sign above my treatment table in my office that shows the progression of how we follow the medication treadmill. From birth to six years of age kids get antibiotics for all ear infections. Remember when I talked about cow's milk and dairy? Well this really increases the incidence of ear infections. I recall a study I read in which a lot of primary care physicians admitted that they gave a mother a prescription for an antibiotic even if doctors knew it was a virus because the mothers asked for "something" since they paid for the office visit. Never mind that there is no cell wall in viruses. The cell wall of bacteria is the structure the antibiotic works on to kill the infection. Yet, some creative doctors rationalized that even if it is a viral infection, it is leaving them more open to contract a bacterial infection. Is this a misguided attempt to justify the creation of super bugs which is happening at an alarming rate today? Back in 1995 the CDC estimated that there were 20 million unnecessary antibiotic prescriptions given for viral infections. TODAY it is many millions more. I recently watched a segment on the evening news that maintained antibiotics are not necessary half of the time. They said patients are more likely to get antibiotics if they expect to during an office visit.

When talking about antibiotics it reminds me of a patient I have who was given the quinolone class of antibiotics which resulted in permanent damage to the muscles and ligaments in his knees. In fact, the patient told me that when the doctor gave him the prescription, he even asked about the side effects which the doctor played down. My patient took his first pill the next morning. By noon he had burning pain in his lower legs to his knees that got progressively worse. He had to crawl out of his office and get help to go to the emergency room. He has had several tendons and ligament ruptures since - all as a result of this class of antibiotics, which he said were not even supposed to be given out anymore. Nor were they supposed to be given out at the time of his prescription according to a class action suit he discovered against the company who developed this drug. Why are doctors still writing prescriptions for it today in 2013? The answer of course is money.

Let's get back to my sign above the adjusting table. For children 4 to 16 years old Ritalin and or Adderall is the drug of choice to keep up good behavior and increase the ability to focus. Both of these have a very good street value now for kids to abuse as a recreational drug. Now the new scare is prescription drug abuse. When the going gets tough with the challenges of adolescence, don't you think the teen is going to just take a drug and make the pain go away? An ad by the Medicine Abuse Project shows that 44% of teens know at least one friend who abuses prescription drugs. By the time they are seniors in high school, 20% of the students will have abused prescription painkillers and 9-10% will have abused tranquilizers, sedatives, and ADHD drugs.

Next, the sign shows young adults sixteen to twenty-four years old are consuming a lot of appetite suppressants and drugs to keep them awake such as no doze and Prozac to keep them happy. These are followed by Xanax to calm them down. Finally, as they reach retirement age, they are programmed take a pill for every ill. The pharmaceutical companies pay billions of dollars a year in advertising to keep people on this drug treadmill-from birth to death. **In fact, for**

every $1 spent on research there is $19 spent on promotion and development.

When we look at drugs we have to look at the primary mechanism behind them. DRUGS SUPRESS SYMPTOMS AND CERTAIN RESPONSES OR REACTIONS in the body. Due to the popularity with NASCAR today in this country, I like to use the analogy of the dashboard in your car representing your brain - both take care of a body. When a warning light comes on in your car, you have two choices: you can either investigate it or ignore it. Investigating it could entail going to a garage and having it looked at by a mechanic. If you choose to ignore it, you could just trace the wire going from the engine to the dashboard and cut it. It will not light up anymore. I liken the second choice to the use of drugs in your body. Now keep in mind that I am not talking about trauma when you know what you did to cause the pain and symptoms you are now suffering from and you just need some relief medication to get through the day or to sleep. I am also not talking about those situations where there is no other option and a particular drug is needed to function. On the contrary, I am talking about those people who have NO CLUE why they are feeling bad. They just want to forget about it, to cut the wire, so to speak. We all know somebody who suddenly dropped dead with no warning because he denied or covered with drugs his warning symptoms. By cutting the wire or taking medications to block symptoms you are really just playing Russian roulette in essence. The body uses symptoms such as pain to tell you, "Hey dummy, there is a problem down here. Investigate its causes." When you just cover these symptoms up the body will create other ones, sometimes not near your current ones, to REALLY try and TELL you that something is wrong.

I want to thank Dr. John Pepelnjak for posting this valuable article on the Johnson forum today from the documentary film "Pill Poppers" written by Dr. Mercola. This is a real eye opener for those who think the drug industry has our best interests at heart. The documentary asks the question, "Are these pills really beneficial or are they doing more harm than good?" Dr. Mercola states some startling facts. For instance, over the course of a person's lifetime, he will have been prescribed 14,000 pills not including over the counter medicines.

Many people are unaware that a new drug is often formed more by serendipity than by science. The documentary begins in a lab at the major drug company GSK (GlaxoSmithKline) that stores 2 million drug compounds in a vault, but know neither their lifesaving nor detrimental effects. A disease molecule is introduced into each of these 2 million substances and researchers then look for any reaction. Some say it is like looking for a needle in a haystack. Further tests are then conducted to find out what happens and why. It costs an estimated $1 billion and takes 15 years to come up with a licensed drug, the "ultimate goal." Now here is the really scary part. More about this licensed drug is known AFTER it is released to the public because that is when the really big numbers of people begin taking it. Clinical trials could never simulate this widespread exposure. So contrary to what most people think, "Just because the drug makes it through the regulatory process, it's no guarantee of safety." Talk about the blind leading the blind; one person in the documentary is quoted as saying, "Drugs are not designed but discovered, and we only find out what they really do to us when we take them." So what would the medical doctors who constantly state that chiropractic is not scientific say to that?

Many of a drug's effects are also found out or discovered by mistake. A lot of people really think that a drug exerts specifically designed effects on certain biological pathways in their bodies. In other words they think this drug knows to go to a certain tissue and only affect that tissue. The reality is that most of a drug's effects are observed and not designed. Just like the manner in which a drug is discovered, it is also labeled. Viagra for example, was an angina medication. It was a "surprise or dumb luck" that it also helped erectile dysfunction. Now if it was a surprise that the drug helps something else wouldn't that lead one to believe that the mechanism is totally unknown and raises even more questions about possible side effects? Are you with me here? Another example of a drug's "dumb luck" is with the ADHD drug, Ritalin. Originally designed for adults with depression, researchers still do not know how it really works, yet and according to Mercola, it is "Already morphing into a drug with another purpose- a study drug." Ventolin inhalers given for Asthma can also prevent premature labor and arsenic poisoning. Now these drugs are making a comeback as a treatment for leukemia?

Along with the dumb luck also come the side effects; no drug is without them. All pill poppers should be aware of this. In the documentary, a GSK spokesperson even said, "When you make a medicine you're trying to alter a fundamental biological process. That's a pretty profound change; you can't do without producing some unwanted side effects-so then the question is, what risks are you prepared to take for what benefit?"

Drug companies even create diseases to fit their proposed treatments. Dr. Mercola maintains that they create non existing diseases and really exaggerate minor ones. The consumers will then rush to their doctors and ask for the medication just like those in the commercials. Again, this is the pill for every ill mentality we are creating for our next generation. Dr. Mercola also states that erectile dysfunction is an occasional problem for many men and that, he says, is normal. But Viagra is marketed in a way that says it is abnormal if a man EVER has the problem. The female sex drive is yet another example of this labeling. Calling it "female sexual dysfunction", drug companies are working for a cure. In order to market its wonder drug

Paxil, GSX hired a marketing company to raise public awareness about how depression is an "under diagnosed disease." There is a disease called "Social Anxiety Disorder" which was previously known as shyness? I was always somewhat shy growing up therefore I find the label for shyness particularly disconcerting. There were TV ads a few years back that asked us to "imagine being allergic to people." Celebrities and psychiatrists promoted this so -called disorder in the media and the mention of social anxiety disorder in the press rose from 50 to 1 billion in just two years. The social anxiety disease became the "third most common mental illness" in America.

Dr. Mercola claims that drug companies are not just trying to treat disease now but also RISK FACTORS. In case anyone may develop a disease in the future, drug companies have drugs to take as a preventative measure. *Some preventative drugs are giving someone side effects to prevent some possible disease that the proposed drug could not help anyway?*

In the last chapter I went over the causes of poor health. Now I want to give you the information that the current medical model of health care recommends. It begins with the recommended diet developed from the so-called "revised food pyramid." In "The Great Cholesterol Con", written in 2006 by Anthony Colpo MD, he explains how the lambasting of cholesterol/fat in our diet originated with the dietary guidelines in 1977. The theories about cholesterol and fat as beneficial were rejected by many scientists due to financial interest. In his book, Colpo also describes the flaws of the S.A.D. and picks apart study after study - of which many of the deemed "high cholesterol" coronary artery disease drug protocols, are based upon today.

Cholesterol is an alcohol and a lipid, or fat; mostly made in the liver but other organs make smaller amounts. It is crucial to the membrane permeability and structure to every cell in your body. This means it is involved in what fluids pass in and out of your cells. It is also the basic substance from which adrenal stress hormones and sex hormones are made. As I said earlier, it gives the red blood cells the ability to squeeze through tighter spaces. Moreover, it coats the nerve cells so the impulses needed for all aspects of life are possible. In fact, it is in the greatest concentration in the brain and nervous system acting as insulation and for nerve conduction. This information is supplied by double blind studies done in the 1990's. While focusing on trying to prove the evils of high cholesterol, researchers actually found that drug induced lower cholesterol levels led to motor skill reduction, depression, and attention span shortening. Cholesterol is an important anti-oxidant. Remember the causes of free radical damage in my "why we are so unhealthy" previous section? Low cholesterol helps increase these free radicals. **The truth is, you could not live without cholesterol.** *Many contend cholesterol is one of the most important substances in our bodies.* The cholesterol quagmire has been a highly debated issue in this country for many years. Perhaps the most known cholesterol study done was the Framingham study in 1948. When the scientific evidence to support high cholesterol as the smoking gun for coronary heart disease was not there, those funding the study found that there was simply too much money invested and too much profit to be made on drug sales to admit they were wrong. Instead they went into denial and misconstrued the results in study after study to suit their needs in supporting the use of lowering cholesterol drugs. To put it simply, researchers let questionable, unproven and even contradictory evidence validate their hypothesis of the evils of cholesterol.

What the Framingham study did find was very interesting. Those with high cholesterol were not dying any faster than controls. In fact those over 50 years old, with higher cholesterol, were living longer than those with lower cholesterol levels. What they found was unexpected. If those taking the cholesterol lowering drugs had fewer heart attacks, it was due to serendipitous effect by reducing inflammation not cholesterol but not without damaging side effects. That was a huge wake-up call right there that indeed **INFLAMMATION** is the key, not cholesterol. Furthermore, despite decades of derogatory statements about what the medical establishment considers "high cholesterol," **I contend that there is no disease called high cholesterol.**

In an article on Dr. Mercola's website, by Dr. Ron Rosedale, titled "Cholesterol is NOT the Cause of Heart Disease," he explains in more detail about the pro-cholesterol studies than I have. I think it deserves a little deeper discussion to satisfy those cholesterol lowering drug supporters. I said earlier that cholesterol is like a band aid when the arteries get inflamed from substances such as sugar and/or nano bacteria liberated when food is cooked. Our bodies are made to eat raw food. This cholesterol then becomes oxidized and goes rancid. Remember free radical damage? It then can damage the artery walls. Again, we have to try to omit whatever causes this inflammation. Research has shown, however, that omega three fats, which are good for us, also can become rancid. But since this book is called "A Common Sensible Approach," is it not common sense to try and prevent the fatty acids and cholesterol from going rancid instead of just not eating them? Dr. Rosedale presents a good analogy. He says that if you use the medical rational for treating Alzheimer's disease, you would just remove the brain so that it would not become diseased!

Low density lipoproteins or LDLs are the most important numbers in the cholesterol controversy that society is so obsessed with. Because of the S.A.D. insulin resistance frequently occurs. What happens is that our diet is so full of sugar the insulin gets resistant and requires more and more before it lets the sugar get in the cells. These LDL particles then become smaller and less dense. Consequently, they can squeeze between the endothelial cells which line the inside of the arteries. This is called the "gap junction" of the endothelium. Here the LDL cholesterol particles can get stuck and potentially oxidize, resulting in inflammation and plaque formation. But we must remember, however, that the LDLs are the transporter of cholesterol and phospholipids to the central nervous system, where they act as fatty insulators. This is important for nerve impulses; it is a conductor for them so they can fire rapidly. In the presence of inorganic "enriched" iron, which I previously discussed, is found in white flour products, the LDLs can be readily oxidized and have been shown to cause cell death. Buildup of this oxidized LDL represents a possible link to neurodegenerative diseases such as ALS (Amyotrophic Lateral Sclerosis).

Dr. Rosedale state that scientific research has shown a definite causal effect of insulin resistance on heart and vascular disease, yet almost all cholesterol studies only show an association and are misleading because an association does not imply a cause.

He maintains that the hormones Insulin's and leptin's, a hormone neurotransmitter produced by fat cells involved in the regulation of appetite, malfunction or improper signaling are the cause of elevated cholesterol, triglycerides, and heart disease. Sugar itself is not the cause of diabetes; it is the way the body is utilizing the sugar. The sugar is just following the directions of the body's metabolism. With the average American eating 140 pounds of sugar a year and tons of white flour- iron laden foods, it is almost impossible for the body to process this sugar without a hitch. The "white death" products not only cause sugar damage to arteries, but cell death as well.

This is why taking away cholesterol will not change the root cause of heart disease. Dr. Rosedale points out that the generals of metabolic communication are insulin and leptin. Until they are communicating normally, the cardiovascular epidemic will continue.

Let's take a closer look at statins, the number one selling drug in this country for lowering serum cholesterol; **since 1996 when they first hit the market, they have made $140 billion in profit and outsold every other drug and continue to do so.** For many years the statin-cholesterol lowering medication mechanism was thought to lower the lower density lipoproteins or LDL portion of cholesterol. These are proteins in the blood which carry the cholesterol from the liver to the cells in tissues throughout the body. Andreas Moritz, author of "The Amazing Liver and Gallbladder Flush" explains how the low density lipoproteins are large cholesterol molecules unlike the smaller high density lipoproteins and cannot pass through blood vessel walls. These LDL cholesterol molecules must be rebuilt in the liver cells, leave the blood stream in the liver, and combine with bile in the small intestine to later be eliminated from the body. Since the S.A.D. promotes gallstone formation and a decrease bile flow, the LDL pathway to exit the liver is often blocked resulting in less bile flowing to remove the toxins with the LDLs. Statin drugs work by blocking an enzyme or protein involved in the synthesis of cholesterol in the liver and do not worry at all about the pathway or exit from the body. But statins also block the production of a very important vitamin - like enzyme naturally found in the body known as Co-Enzyme Q10. Low levels of this have a huge negative impact on cardiovascular health because this enzyme prevents LDLs from oxidizing. Depleted Co-enzyme Q10 is very harmful to you.

Statins also have ramifications of blocking more down-stream or later occurring necessary reactions your body would normally have. Remember that hormones, enzymes, and etc., substances have more than one job and their effects are far reaching. If you block one substance doing its duty, you may be blocking 5-10 other processes which should occur down the line. This is a first-hand example of the unpredictability of far reaching adverse effects of statin drugs.

I must emphasize about the acknowledged side effects of statin drugs. The most common are: muscle aches and pains, lethargy or extreme tiredness, memory loss, depression, and digestive complaints. Here are some symptoms you may have when your Co-Enzyme Q10 is deficient: heart attack, congestive heart failure, hair loss, gum disease, cancer, angina, and high blood pressure. I remember in the early 2000s when patients would complain of a lot of increased musculoskeletal pain without any known cause. I would ask them about statin drugs and they would say, "Yeah, I am on Lipitor." I asked myself why are so many of these patients, with increased muscle pain and no plausible explanations, on statins. When patients questioned their medical doctor about muscle pain as a side effect of a statin, their doctors were quick to reply, "It is rare and happens in about 3% of cases." There are 45-50 million Americans taking statins which equates to about twice the number who go to a Chiropractor. Remember only 7% of the population goes to a Chiropractor. How many patients coming to us chiropractors for back pain may actually have their symptoms brought on by gluten, the mycoplasma infection or STATINS. Numerous patients have told me that "the pain just came on" and that they do not "remember doing anything physical that may have brought the pain on." Other side effects of statin use are episodes of amnesia, termed TGA or total global amnesia which can last from hours to days plus memory loss. Sometimes long-term memory loss is found along with disorientation. Fortunately, this side effect discontinues after one discontinues his or her statin intake. I must also mention the correlation of testosterone and statin use. Statins inhibit the enzyme required for cholesterol synthesis; the downstream effect is a reduction in any hormones that are made with cholesterol as the starting material. Testosterone is one of those hormones and is reduced with statin intake. We see so many of low testosterone ads on television that advocate statins to reduce your cholesterol, which inadvertently lowers your testosterone, and testosterone cream to raise your testosterone levels? In effect, your testes will stop producing its own testosterone since you are rubbing it in from an exogenous source. You know the drug company's response to this scenario will be that such a low dose of statins will do nothing to the testosterone production. Moreover, the drug spokesman will add, these patients have a disease called "high cholesterol" which is far more risky than low testosterone levels and there is a drug for that anyway. This is just an example of the logic you will encounter with the medical doubletalk justifying many drugs. An incorrect premise will lead to an incorrect conclusion. So you can easily see how facts need to be BASED ON LOGIC and not partial truths. Here is an example from my freshman philosophy class. All fish have fins. Whales have fins. Therefore whales are fish. It is the art of using the language and of partial truths. You see mom and dad; I did learn something in college.

Keep in mind that when they conduct a clinical trial, researchers exclude many conditions that are in the general population in any random sample. They are left with a healthier study sample that is not representative of the general public. There is also something called the "washout period" during the drug study or clinical trial when any subject having side effects is dismissed. Researchers claim they are sparing the dismissed subjects from any further side effects. Logic should tell us that they just want to downplay side effects.

My purpose is to demonstrate why we are so sick and to present a common sensible approach to be healthier. If you think about it, the multimillion statin prescriptions depict the faulty premises of researchers who believe that because a person's serum levels of a certain substance are not within the arbitrary range set by a committee in the medical establishment are questionable and of deep concern to say the least. Arguably, the research is not there to support these prescriptions-this is sort of like the "fuzzy math" that George W. Bush was often accused of using.

Saturated fat has also taken a beating over the years. The 1900s brought about the theory of saturated fat leading to coronary heart disease. Countless studies from that time into the present showing correlation between saturated fat and coronary heart disease continue. However, a researcher by the name of Ancel Keys made it his life's mission to find the negative correlation saturated fat consumption has to coronary heart disease. His major study was ridiculed by the World Health Organization, so he came up with another "seven countries study," which seemed to only use data from studies that supported his hypothesis and ignored the other data that contradicted it. Unbelievably, it was accepted and was to change the course of modern medicine concerning saturated fat intake. The studies we were never privy to were the ones supporting the opposite position that lower levels of saturated fat levels led to an increase in coronary heart disease and stroke. The famous cholesterol study I just previously mentioned, "The Framingham Study" actually showed that the people who ate the most saturated fat and cholesterol were also the people who ate the most food, were the most active, and who weighed the least. Not surprisingly, it also found these people had the lowest serum cholesterol. The Framingham study supported saturated fat.

Do you see a trend here that maybe much of the information we have been told about diet and healthy nutrition has been MISINFORMATION? Remember, the drug companies want you to just follow the herd on the medication/hospital/death treadmill that supports their multibillion dollar industry. But if you look at the logic, or better yet, the holes in their logic, it is really quite easy to expose the enumerable flawed studies that are continually presented.

Depression is a major complaint of a majority of twenty year old plus females who come into my office. According to their charts, over 90% of them are on a mood enhancer such as Prozac, Zoloft, and Elavil. In a great article written by Adam Hadhazy on Feb 12, 2010 entitled- "Think twice: How the Guts 'Second Brain' influences Mood and Well Being," he explains the connection between these mood enhancing drugs and digestive health. Although, this is a complicated subject I will try not to be too technical. I want to emphasize how important good digestion is in terms of mental health as well as overall health. The author brings up how we feel "butterflies" in the stomach before a sporting event. There is a huge network of neurons lining our guts. It is so extensive that some scientists have dubbed the gut our "second brain." Everybody agrees however, that there is no conscious decision making by the second brain. Activities like religious debate, poetry, and various philosophies are left to the brain in the head.

Adam Hadhazy mentions a great book written by Michael Gershon in 1998 in fact called *"The Second Brain."* He is chairman of the Department of Anatomy and Cell Biology at New York-Presbyterian Hospital/Columbia University Medical Center. And, he is an expert in the field of neurogastroenterology, or how the nervous system interacts with the digestive system." This network of neural or nerve tissue in the gut is nine meters long from end to end from the esophagus to the anus and contains more than 100 million neurons. This is more than either the spinal cord or the peripheral (outside of the brain and spine) nervous system. It is filled with neurotransmitters- the same ones I discussed earlier. In fact, 95% of the body's serotonin- the feel-good neurotransmitter, is found in the bowels and not in the brain. This led many to believe that the gut does much more than simply handle digestive duties. It indicates that, "the little brain in our innards connected to the big one in our skulls, partly determines our mental state and plays key roles in certain diseases throughout the body." Let me explain this further.

"The system is way too complicated to have evolved only to make sure things come out of your colon," says Emeran Mayer, professor of physiology, psychiatry, and behavioral sciences at the U.C.L.A. School of medicine. Scientists were shocked to discover that 90% of the fibers of the vagus nerve- the major visceral nerve, carries information from the gut to the brain and not the other way around. "Some of that information is unpleasant according to Gershon."

Let's go back to the butterflies in our stomach. This is component of the gut signaling a physiological stress response, according to Gershon. However, he says it is but one example; even though digestive upset can sour one's mood, everyday wellbeing may rely on messages from the brain below to the brain above. An example, of this is using electric stimulation of the vagus nerve, which mimics these signals. By the way, this is a current treatment for depression.

Given the connection between the two brains, if you will, depression treatments that target the mind can unintentionally impact the gut. The enteric (gut) nervous system and the brain use more than 30 neurotransmitters. Because the antidepressant meds-the selective serotonin uptake inhibitors- (SSRIs) increase serotonin levels, it is no mystery that medications meant to cause chemical changes in the mind also provoke digestive issues as a side effect. Irritable Bowel Syndrome, affecting over 2 million Americans, is also a result of too much serotonin in our gut. This could be called mental illness of the gut.

In support of the gut influencing the brain, I must mention another article discussing probiotics heralded as the new Prozac. Probiotics are bacteria which benefit the host and are found in fermented foods like yogurt and sauerkraut. According to cutting edge research, they may be able to combat depression and anxiety. UCLA researchers reported that a MRI (Magnetic Resonance Imaging) study confirmed certain areas of the brain, which regulate emotions and internal body sensations, were altered in women who ate probiotic yogurt regularly. They used an emotional reactivity test, for example, by showing test women pictures of angry scared faces. The women who ate the probiotics showed a decrease in activity in the corresponding brain areas according to neuropsychiatrist Daniel Amen MD, a brain mapping specialist. Women who did not eat the probiotics had stable or increased activity in these same areas. The study consisted of 36 women and was published in the Journal of Gastroenterology.

Dr. Kirsten Tillsch, associate professor of medicine at UCLA's David Geffen School of Medicine and lead author of the study wrote, "When we consider the implications of this work, the old saying 'you are what you eat' and 'gut feelings' take on new meaning." A New Zealand psychology researcher is so enthusiastic about these findings that he is launching a new study, which will consist of 80 patients with depression, who will receive probiotic supplements for four months.

Another study published online in New Medicine on February 7, 2010, showed that if serotonin release from the gut was inhibited in post-menopausal rats, it counteracted the bone-deteriorating disease osteoporosis. Gerald Karsenty, the lead author of the study and chairman of the Department of Genetics at Columbia University said, "It was totally unexpected that the gut would regulate bone mass to the extent that one could use this regulation to cure -at least in rodents- osteoporosis."

Gershon also discovered that the serotonin in the second brain might be related to autism, the developmental disorder often first noticed in childhood. He found that genes involved in neuron synapses, a structure that allows a nerve cell to pass a chemical or electrical signal to another cell in the brain, are also involved in the gut neuronal synapses. He stated that if these genes are affected in autism it could explain why so many kids with autism have digestive abnormalities in addition to the elevated serotonin levels in their gut.

This of course is reinforcing how important it is to keep the gastrointestinal or digestive system optimally functioning so the brain and the rest of the body can also be optimally functioning. When talking about the rampant depression afflicting so many in this country, we must also bear in mind the importance of the brain thyroid connection.

There are many good books written on the thyroid gland. Dr. Michael Johnson, the leader of the Neurometaboliic group, just published with his own thyroid book called, *"You can beat Thyroid disorders naturally."* I will not provide much detail here but will just mention that the thyroid gland influences energy levels, moods and emotions mostly due to altered blood sugar levels. Let me explain.

When blood sugar is normal, your body is running like a well fueled race car. But when it spikes and dives, it runs like a car on bad gas that is sputtering and stalling. People who consume the S.A.D. are eating at a highly processed, white sugar, salt and flour, nutrient-lacking smorgasbord. This makes your blood sugar levels dance up and down like Beyoncé at the 2013 Super Bowl, and is known as blood sugar dysregulation. When you finish eating a typical American fast food meal, for example, your body has to process large amounts sugar. Keep in mind now that I am talking about all of the food you eat, not just literally sugar- based foods like dessert for example. Your body must break everything you eat down to the simple sugar glucose so it burns it as energy. When this meal is broken down the sugar is floating around in your bloodstream trying to get into the cells. The problem is that from constantly eating this type of diet, your cells have grown insensitive to the receptors that usually signal them to open up. I am talking about Insulin sensitivity and particularly insulin resistance. To review, Insulin is a hormone that is made in the pancreas, whose job is to get the glucose in the cells. Your pancreas must secrete a lot of insulin to get the sugar from this typical sugary meal into the cells. After a while, however, the cells are already full of glucose. Now even more insulin is released trying to get every last bit of glucose into the cells. This creates insulin resistance and signals the brain to say, "Get me some more fuel... eat more." As a result, we eat even more sugar. This cycle continues over and over. When you cannot get the glucose into the cells, you start to get brain fog and feelings of unpleasantness; this can lead to mood swings and depression because your brain is THE MOST VORACIOUS USER OF GLUCOSE. With this insulin resistance- when the glucose cannot get into the cells because the cells are already full, the glucose then circulates around the body wreaking havoc on the interior of the arteries and eventually is turned into triglycerides or fats. This process uses a lot of energy, which results in the post meal "carb coma." This applies to you if you always find yourself napping after eating. As you can see, this blood sugar teeter totter most of this country is on is a perfect situation for chronic fatigue syndrome or low energy state which easily leads to depression. It can also lead to metabolic syndrome, a precursor to adult onset Type II diabetes. The pancreas, which manufactures the insulin, becomes tired and Type II diabetes is born. New research indicates that the neurodegenerative disease Alzheimer's is really just Type III Diabetes. Suzanne de la Monte, a researcher from Rhode Island Hospital found that Alzheimer's progresses as the brain develops a resistance to insulin, which leads to improper metabolism of fats. This then leads to chronic toxic inflammation. Thus, lipid or fat metabolism must be restored in order to reverse this damage. Here lies a major problem. So many elderly patients diagnosed with Alzheimer's are also on statin cholesterol lowering drugs, known to increase the incidence of BOTH ALZHEIMERS AND DIABETES. I just talked about these drugs in the last section. The elderly with Alzheimer's and depression are an increasingly a major concern. Many people do not realize how many baby boomers are AARP ages now. Pennsylvania for example, is only second to Florida for the oldest population in the US.

If the general practitioner writes the patient a prescription for Zoloft, for example, he may have some relief for weeks or months, the manner in which most medications work on any symptoms. Soon, however, the body gets accustomed to the medication's proposed mechanism of action and accommodates for it usually by providing the person with either stronger symptoms or another symptom altogether. Your brain is telling you, "Hey dummy, there is a problem here that needs dealing with. Don't just cover up the warning signs and go about your business and hope for the best." In light of our previous, "second brain" discussion, it's no surprise we see predominantly gastrointestinal side effects such as nausea and diarrhea when looking up Zoloft. But then there are also serious nervous system side effects such as insomnia. This makes sense since adequate amounts of the neurotransmitter dopamine, which are needed for sleep, are also found in the gut.

I also need to discuss drug interaction problems. Let's go back to the depression topic. Today there are so many people on antidepressants- in fact about 1 in 10 Americans. This is a 400% increase in the use of anti-depressants over the past two decades. The drug interaction I am referring to occurs when a person on antidepressants takes anti-inflammatories at the same time. Who may this be? Many of the same patients suffering from depression are the ones suffering from arthritis- usually the elderly. The selective serotonin re-uptake inhibitors, the category that many of the common antidepressants fall into, work by injuring glial cells which are nerve cells. The antidepressant will accumulate in the glial cells and cause- ready for this: **a highly inflammatory toxic response.** This then triggers the release of another substance known as BDNF (brain derived neurotrophic factor), which is one of the most important healing compounds in your brain. Nerve cells, when injured, have to either fix themselves or have a strategy to develop new nerve growth and cannot just split and divide like other cells in your body can. Thus the mechanism of these SSRIs is to injure the nerve cells by inducing CHRONIC TOXIC INFLAMMATION- the same that causes pretty much every chronic disease, and this will then trigger the release of BDNF to fix it. *Now you can understand why taking anti-inflammatories will interfere with this process.* Those people with the lowest BDFN levels also have the most severe depression. Also, people with thyroid problems cannot properly activate this compound. When you remember what I recently said about the second brain and serotonin levels, it is easy to see why the elderly are so prone to gastrointestinal complications. In fact, the elderly have a 1 in 4,000 risk of death from gastrointestinal complications. Can you see how this information is all related? Again, depressed people have run out of BDNF. Their high stress levels depleted it. By giving them SSRIs, you are giving them a temporary Band-Aid fix that is really an excitotoxic brain injury; not to mention how it also affects the gut.

Proton pump inhibitors, such as Prilosec and Nexium, form another huge drug industry in this country since they are among the most used drugs for G.E.R.D., also known as gastro-esophageal reflux disease. Here are some startling facts about these drugs that you may not have heard. I explained earlier what usually happens with reflux and indigestion. The medical profession places most upper GI problems in the GERD category and prescribes these drugs. There are alarming reports of children suffering stomach complaints leaving a doctor's office with a prescription for one of these drugs. I find these prescriptions unethical. No stomach acid means a lack of methyl groups, which may lead to a chronic disease after long use.

I will now discuss some dangerous facts about proton pump inhibitors. Long-term use of five years increases risk of hip fractures, and 7 or more years of use increases significant risk of osteoporotic fractures. In fact, postmenopausal woman have 3.5 times the incidence of vertebral fractures if they use the drugs long-term. I already discussed the need for minerals as a foundation for bone health and that we cannot get them from the soil anymore. There are reports associating low calcium and magnesium levels due to proton pump inhibitor use with extreme muscular weakness of the arms and legs, to hypoparathyroidism, and swallowing disorders. The low stomach acid as a result of these drugs also is a breeding ground for yeast, parasites, and bacteria. In fact, by taking them you increase the chances of salmonella and campylobacter by a factor of 2.5. With drugs like the proton pump inhibitors this acidic stomach pH is taken away, enabling H pylori to thrive causing peptic ulcers and stomach inflammation. Less known, however, is the fact that H pylori will even destroy the blood vessels to the heart. Autopsies are currently revealing H pylori in lesions of stroke and heart attack victims. Low stomach acid can also be a contributing factor to heart attacks and strokes. As a matter of fact undigested proteins, due to the use of proton pump inhibitors, become absorbed and then stimulate an allergic reaction in the body which may lead to auto-immunity; this happens when the body attacks itself. In addition, these drugs stimulate the TH2 aspect of your immune system, increasing the incidence of food allergies. I talked about this is detail with leaky gut earlier. Proton pump inhibitors also impair the stomach's ability to produce Vit B12 causing a deficiency that can lead to B12 anemia.

Ironically, the most common side effects of these drugs are STOMACH PAIN. **Look at how illogical this is. Give a patient a drug for stomach pain which causes stomach pain, is no more effective than a placebo, and causes mineral depletion and protein malabsorption, and will cause osteoporosis.** Moreover, the diagnosis for which these drugs are often given is usually not even the correct diagnosis for many patients. Eosinophilic esophagitis has no known agreed upon cause but has been attributed to "allergies" from toxic mold spores in our living and working environment. Over the past twenty-five years those wrongly diagnosed with GERD actually have eosinophilic esophagitis and no reflux at all. To recognize this would eliminate the need for the billion dollars pharmaceutical bonanza from selling proton pump inhibitors. Thus any further discussion of eosinophilic esophagitis in many medical journals has been suppressed.

For those that complain they have too much stomach acid, the stomach is well equipped to handle the most acidic pH with no problem at all. Those who may risk damage from too much stomach acid, however, are people **also** taking aspirin, other non-steroidal anti-inflammatory drugs, or those on Prednisone which weakens the stomach wall. Consequently, the body's tolerance for the acidic environment of the stomach is lowered. Not only do we have the antidepressants and anti-inflammatories but also the statins and proton pump inhibitors are adding damage.

Speaking of aspirin, you cannot watch anything on television without seeing ads promoting this "wonder drug" aspirin; as part of an everyday regimen to combat heart disease. Well it is about time people heard the truth about the research behind taking an aspirin a day to thin the blood. In an excellent recent summary of the major studies done on aspirin and its ability to prevent strokes and heart disease, published in the JAMA, (Journal of the American Medical Association) researchers found no benefit to taking an aspirin a day in preventing heart disease. They concluded that those taking daily aspirin and Ibuprofen regularly, actually double their risk of a fatal heart attack. There are thousands of people dying each year from side effects of aspirin; these include gastrointestinal bleeding and hemorrhagic strokes which constitutes about 20% of all strokes. Taking daily aspirin can actually cause a formation of a blood clot, rather than prevent it. This contradiction sounds familiar, doesn't it? Another JAMA study, in 2010 by Fawkes, et al., found that aspirin gave zero protection against all-cause mortality. Specifically, it said there was zero protection when taking an aspirin per day for such things as: initial fatal or non-fatal heart attack, initial stroke, and TIA (transient ischemic attack). This study did find though, that the aspirin per day group was 70% more likely to be hospitalized for an initial major hemorrhage. A study by Ogawah, et al: In JAMA November 2008 looked at taking low dose aspirin in order to prevent atherosclerosis in patients with Type II or sugar diabetes. The article was really studying how low dose aspirin would prevent cardiovascular events in these patients. The conclusion showed no reduction in heart attacks or stroke. In a study by Ridkerpm, et al., in the New England Journal of Medicine in March 2005, female subjects in a randomized trial were given low dose aspirin an attempt to prevent heart attacks and strokes. Here the conclusion showed no decrease in heart attacks, but there was a slight decrease of ischemic stroke, however, this was offset by an increase in hemorrhagic strokes.

What is even more amazing about aspirin is that it has been known for at least **twenty years** that daily low dose aspirin does not protect you from a heart attack or stroke. A study in Australia in the Medical Tribune on June 25, 1992, found that patients who had some blockage in arteries going to the brain were three times more likely to have a stroke if they were taking low dose aspirin- even from as little as a half a tablet per day. The original study, by the AMA known as the "Physician's Health Study" declared that low dose aspirin will decrease the incidence of a second heart attack. The problem with this study and the reduced risk of a second heart attack finding is that the participants were not only taking aspirin but also supplementing with Magnesium- the important trace mineral I discussed earlier. What the study also showed was that with the decreased heart attacks there was an equal increase in strokes. So the overall mortality rate of people taking the buffered aspirin versus controls was unchanged. To summarize, there was a slight heart attack decrease which was due to the magnesium, but the incidence of strokes increased.

A British study appeared a short time later that tried to confirm the "Physician's Health Study", but they omitted the magnesium. Their conclusion was that low dose daily aspirin did absolutely nothing as far as lowering the incidence of heart attacks. Ironically, the subjects in this study suffered from such severe gastrointestinal bleeding that many of them had to drop out.

Research at the University of California, and appearing in the British Medical Journal found that elderly people taking aspirin daily almost doubled their chances of ischemic heart disease. Other findings of this study were: an increased incidence of colon and kidney cancers, an increased death rate from hemorrhagic stroke, along with an increase in diseases due to bleeding ulcers and intestinal bleeding. Thus you should research this topic on your own and not just the television commercials. <u>Don't drink the Kool- Aid.</u> The advertising campaign for aspirin has been very effective regardless of how cheap the drug is.

Blood pressure pills are another huge problem in our country. According to the CDC, it is estimated that one third of Americans suffer from high blood pressure and more than half do not have it under control. High blood pressure is defined as the systolic or upper number over 140 mm Hg and the lower number or diastolic over 90 mm Hg. Systolic or the upper number is measuring the pressure in the artery when the heart beats. The diastolic pressure or the lower number is measuring the pressure in the artery between heart beats. Pre hypertension is anything more than 120 mm Hg for the systolic and anything greater than 80 mm Hg for the diastolic. In 2005 this normal pressure reading scale changed to 110/70. The 120/80 was always the normal reading up to this point. Some contended that this lowering of the normal values was a response to some of the effects revealed in the massive hormone replacement therapy study involving 27,000 nurses. The study was stopped in 2004 due the fact that too many women were having strokes, heart attacks and breast cancer. This study is known as the "study that discredited hormone replacement therapy." Articles have been written since, on how this study was flawed, but the damage had already been done to Big Pharma. So now you have 40 million women who were taking hormone replacement therapy that were scared off. Speculation is that Big pharma had to make up for lost income somehow. Thus the blood pressure values were lowered which gave credence to adding an additional 1/3 of Americans on blood pressure meds. If you do the math, this makes up for the 40 million women on hormone replacement therapy. To make matters worse, a recent article in The New York Times suggested that as many as 100 million people who thought they were at risk for heart disease may not have been at risk at all. In 2003 when the National Committee on Blood Pressure Prevention met, they decided that relatively low blood pressure readings were a risk for heart disease. Dr. Mercola explains how they "Acknowledged the new affliction- dubbed- prehypertension- didn't necessarily require a need for medication." However, as the New York Times reported, The National Committee on Blood Pressure Prevention still urged doctors to "take high blood pressure more seriously and treat it more aggressively, often with more than one drug." Here is where the 45 million new drug prescriptions came from. This is very similar to what happened in 2001 with statins when the National Lung, Heart, and Blood Institute lowered the cholesterol level guidelines. The committee that came up with guidelines asked for "aggressive treatment" with statins and categorized the need for 23 million prescriptions for statins. Interestingly enough, eight of the nine authors of these guidelines had financial ties to statin makers. For years, the New York Times newspaper continues to condemn the practice of doctors in study trials run by pharmaceutical companies receiving huge payments from them.

I think Dr. Mercola says it best: "It's hard to guess how many people since then have been taking blood pressure drugs and statins unnecessarily just because their doctors chose to treat them aggressively. But what's criminal is that these are just two examples of how drug companies can boost sales by covertly influencing how normally benign conditions are defined and treated."

We cannot omit prescription pain medications such as oxycodone and Percocet out of this topic. **After all, Americans consume 80% of the world's supply of painkillers every year.** This is more than 110 tons of opiates as the country's prescription drug epidemic explodes. It is enough to give every American 64 Vicodin or Percocets. I will talk more about this prescription epidemic later.

Of great concern are the Non-steroidal anti-inflammatories such as Advil and Tylenol. There are 17 million Americans who use NSAIDS on a daily basis for headaches, arthritis, sore muscles, and just about every type of pain you could imagine. These drugs work by blocking prostaglandins, which are hormone-like substances that irritate nerve endings and cause pain sensations. Some of the side effects from their constant use are dangerous, and many people do not realize this because medical doctors downplay them. Let's look at the liver, whose function I have already described in detail. Taking NSAIDS can really harm this organ. You can suffer from drug induced inflammation of the liver or hepatitis, and elevated liver enzymes. Usually these two conditions can be reversed if you just stop taking the drugs. What is more serious however, are two other conditions; vanishing bile duct syndrome, whose cause is linked to the NSAID Ibuprofen, which DESTROYS the bile duct and acute liver failure. This occurs in a short time and is mostly a risk for heavy NSAID users and those who are heavy alcohol users as well. Unfortunately, these two latter conditions can result in the need for a liver transplant. Heavy NSAID users who take a handful daily, at the first sign of jaundice or a yellowing of the skin and whites of the eyes, itching, dark urine, or right upper quadrant pain below the nipple line- please get yourself to the emergency room ASAP.

I tried to cover the major medical complaints by today's society and a few of the most common drugs prescribed. I hope it was not too technical and that I did not get off on too many tangents but I considered it necessary. Of course, I have only touched the surface here but the purpose of this book is not to be technical focusing on the complex science of symptoms, side effects, and drug interactions. I want you to come away from this chapter knowing what you are getting when you go into the medical machine. **Remember, with trauma or lifesaving ability-** *the medical profession shines like no other.* But when it comes to chronic health conditions, it simply misses the mark badly. The country's health is slipping away as a result. The economy is more of a priority than the health of the country, and drug companies put a lot of pressure on the medical doctors to prescribe the current drug that they just spent millions of dollars on to patent. Many of the studies have usually been tailored to make the drug look better than it was in clinical trials. For example, a very small trial may yield a 33% increase in the drug's effectiveness or the same decrease but there may be no mention of the tiny sample size.

Speaking of improper study methodology, I often hear people telling how a recent study denied any health benefit from Vitamin E supplementation. In fact, a 2004 study actually showed higher death rates for those who took 400IUs or more of Vit E daily. Another more recent study stated that daily Vit E supplementation had no benefit whatsoever and did not protect men from prostate cancer. **What they failed to mention, however, is that the researchers only used one form of Vit E: dl- alpha tocopherol, which is the synthetic form. The "dl" signifies that it was synthesized from coal tar derivatives.**

This synthetic form of alpha tocopherol is the "gold standard" when conducting research. It has no antioxidant activity and cannot get into the mitochondria of the cell but only into the bloodstream. Therefore it is not effective and should be discarded. This d alpha tocopherol is the most common form of Vitamin E in dietary supplements, but it is the **gamma tocotrienols form that is one of the most powerful antioxidants known to man.** There are eight naturally occurring forms of Vit E which make Vit E complete. You not only have the alpha tocopherol, but also gamma, delta, and beta forms; then there are the tocotrienols. There are alpha, gamma, beta, and delta tocotrienols. All of these together make the Vit E complete. PRL uses a natural-live source containing all eight of these.

And any derogatory or damaging information making the drug look bad is usually left out of most studies. One pharmaceutical sales rep told me how he would do "lunch and learns" three to four days a week. He would go to a medical doctor's office and bring gourmet catered lunches for the staff and doctors. While they were eating, he would lecture about the latest and greatest new drug. Most of the time the staff would not even be listening he said, but they liked the food and perks. Thus, the lunch and learn drug was the one the doctor would push. There are also articles revealing that some drug companies even promise to pay the doctor's student loans off if they use their brand exclusively!

Many of my patients over the years would say that they were going to their medical doctors to get a second opinion or to see what he would offer. When they said, "He'd better not just offer me drugs." When you go to a butcher does he offer you broccoli and tell you to be a vegetarian? What do you think he is going to do?" In other words most medical doctor's main method of treatment is drugs.

I was studying the Neurometaboliic Forum recently and I found an article by a surgeon Dr. Dwight Lundell in a Health & Wellness publication, March 1, 2012. I still cannot believe a medical doctor, no less a surgeon, wrote this. Chiropractors on our forum have been touting the contents of this one article for years. The surgeon aptly summarized the metabolic aspects of our philosophy. He carefully explains how he actually sees the proof of the medical field's misguided nutritional advice. I am planning a cliff notes version because everything I have explained previously, and believe coheres with the contents of this article.

Dr. Lundell initially agrees that the medical profession made a mistake when it said high cholesterol and saturated fat were the cause of blood vessel damage which led to many of the heart attack and stroke deaths over the past 25 years. Today, these bleak heart attack and stroke death rate statistics have not changed for the better. The following is a quote from Dr. Lundell: *"Despite the facts that 25% of the population takes expensive statin medications, and that fact that we have, reduced the fat content of our diets, more Americans will die this year of heart disease than ever before".* As I may have mentioned earlier, 75 million Americans have heart disease; 57 million are pre-diabetic or have metabolic syndrome X, and 30 million are diabetic. Every year the age afflicted gets younger. He basically said the medical profession's egos got in the way and I concur. With the new research that found "inflammation" the key to all of this pathology, the inferior recommendations on lowering cholesterol are "no longer scientific or morally defensible." This is an amazing admonition because only years before, it was a matter of heresy and could even result in malpractice if a doctor deviated from the standard care recommendations. He continues to say that when there is no inflammation, cholesterol can freely roam about the body and the levels will be whatever is needed. It is inflammation that traps the cholesterol. I explained this previously. Inflammation is usually the first stage of healing in our bodies. Acute inflammation brings about macrophages which are white blood cells that help fight the infection if there is one. Also, it attacks any foreign invaders if there is one. However, due to the S.A.D. and the other problems I have previously mentioned, the inflammation in our bodies can become chronic- long lasting. Dr. Lundell says it well when he stated that chronic inflammation is as bad as acute inflammation is beneficial. It is true that statin drugs have been shown to lower inflammation but, in my opinion, it is not worth the aforementioned side effects.

Dr. Lundell goes on to tell how it is his belief that the S.A.D recommendations, i.e. low saturated fat-high polyunsaturated fat, high carbohydrate diet, has for years been causing "Repeated injury to blood vessels" leading to chronic inflammation and eventually heart disease, diabetes, stroke, and obesity.

Dr. Lundell has had the privilege of seeing thousands of arteries from the inside. "They looked like you took a wire brush and kept scraping them time after time, year after year." He said to visualize what the skin on the outside of your body would look like after years of rubbing a stiff brush against it; it would look like a bloody bruised infected mess. What is the largest contributor or cause of this damage? SUGAR, a highly processed carbohydrate along with white flour and white salt, in the millions of processed foods made from them. One of the best examples is Starbucks's sugary drinks combined with the sweet rolls that go with them, containing the junk oils. These are the polyunsaturated fats he refers to.

He continues to explain how inflammation is inflammation. It does not matter if it is on the inside of your body or the outside; it uses the same mechanism of trying to heal resulting in scarring. Although I already talked about a lot of this, I am repeating some of Dr. Lundell's material because he says it so well, as if he read my mind. "Foods loaded with sugars and simple carbohydrates, or processed with omega-6 oils for long shelf life have been the mainstay of the

American diet for six decades. These foods have been slowly poisoning everyone." As I write these words it is therapeutic to have all that I have believed on this subject for the past years validated.

Dr. Lundell explains how the sweet roll people desire so much really affects your blood sugar levels and how this turns into diabetes. Finally, he mentions that this processed sugar loaded food is soaked in the omega 6 junk oils, which adversely affect the ideal recommended omega 3 to omega 6 ratio. I love this article.

This past Sunday while I was writing the previous pages, the National Geographic channel offered a special about Charles Darwin and the Galapagos islands, showing his journey around the islands, making discoveries which led to his writing of *"The Origin of Species."* It also explained how birds, for example, from different islands not very far apart looked very different as if the birds were different species. One bird, for example, had a longer beak due to the trees having thicker bark on one island versus another. In another comparison of two turtles from different islands, one had a higher shell so that he could lift his head up higher to get food from the higher trees on his island. Why is this relevant to our discussion you ask? The animals had to physically change or adapt to survive in their environment. On the other hand, humans made a conscious decision, urged by advertisers and status ranking to eat all of the grains and processed foods which began to fill the shelves in the early twentieth century markets. People looked to the easier food preparation and changed their dietary habits. The problem is, epigenetically speaking; we will also have to change our DNA by less exposure to toxicity in our environment. The convenience, flavor, and easy food preparation must be substituted for a diet that I will discuss later in another chapter. Nobody forced us to start eating this processed garbage.

I leave this chapter with a few quotes from a very smart medical man. According to Hippocrates, the father of modern medicine, "Our food should be our medicine and our medicine should be our food." The sad thing is, he also said to do no harm in the Hippocratic Oath that all medical doctors must take before they see patients. From the stats on medical mishaps you can see that this piece of advice is not always followed. Also here is an anonymous quote that sums it all up: "The pharmaceutical industry does not create cures but they create customers."

<u>CHAPTER NINE</u>

A Natural Approach to Health

If we look at the word "health", most people would say it means feeling good. But if you look at the WHO (World Health Organization's) definition it is as follows: "Health is state of social, physical, and mental wellbeing and not simply the absence of disease or infirmity." Obviously, I am a chiropractic doctor and all services we offer here at my facility are natural, drug free, and of course surgery free. The name of the facility is Gildea Health and Wellness. As I stated in the beginning of this book, I had an epiphany a couple years ago when I first discovered Dr. Mike Johnson and his Neurometabolic group. Over the past two years I then received my certification in functional nutrition.

Since then my practice has evolved and continues to evolve in order to offer patients the most cutting edge treatments. With all of the research out there really none of us in the healing arts can afford to sit idle and not push for more answers to the chronic disease/health challenge puzzle. Thus I will explain the treatment I offer from A to Z. Keep in mind that my goal is to be able to help anyone who wishes to become healthier; all allow them to see that symptoms alone are not the gauge of health. Again, we all have heard the story of the young person who suddenly dropped dead; although up until that time he felt great and had no history of any physical complaints. It happens, however, that many people have had symptoms, the best motivator to investigate what is wrong, but they often take the path of least resistance and deny them.

Since I have a chiropractic office, of course most people calling for my services involve some type of musculoskeletal pain. Being a chiropractor for twenty five years, I know that this is what most people associate me with. I hope to change this to an association with "total health" in the near future. With many of my patients on arthritis medicine or painkillers for years I will discuss the natural options we have to not only treat the symptoms but also to heal the tissues.

The truth is, we chiropractors are well known for treating neck and back conditions; in fact, we get far superior results over most physical therapists treating neck and back pain as well as neck and lower back disc problems. I will explain why in a later chapter. Furthermore, when dealing with these musculoskeletal complaints I have kept up with the latest and greatest technology to keep my treatment arsenal highly stocked. The use of decompression therapy is nothing new; the Egyptians used archaic traction thousands of years ago for neck and back pain, and the pain radiating down the arms and legs caused most often by disc lesions. Obviously the method of traction has been much more refined over the years. I will explain in detail about this incredible therapy which plays an integral role, in my office, every day getting people better. My most recent piece of technology is the new Cube 4 K-LASER, truly is ahead of its time, and is based on Einstein's quantum mechanics and the photoelectric effect. This therapy can treat many musculoskeletal conditions and actually heals the injured areas. The New York Yankees use it to treat their athletes; you know it must be the real deal.

Energy medicine is another treatment I use in my treatment box with the NanoSRT. The "SRT" stands for stress reduction therapy, the new frontier in today's arsenal against chronic disease, based on Chinese medicine. With this, we use acupuncture principles of energy and light flowing through meridians. Incredibly the exact location of these meridians or energy channels along the body were discovered over 3,000 years ago and are proven to be extremely accurate by today's technology. I am not an acupuncturist and therefore do not engage in "needle acupuncture." Rather, I use a laser light instead to bring about the desired therapeutic effects. This is a fascinating subject that I have researched and studied for about five years. I will explain in detail and how I incorporate the NanoSRT it into my practice later in the book because it holds the answers for many who suffer from food, environmental, animal, and chemical sensitivities to name a few. There is a website for the NanoSRT with a 4 minute video that does an excellent job explaining it in detail; the website is www.NanoSRTsrt.bio.com.

I will save the nutritional component, an addition to my practice, and the most important aspect of total health for last. One day, in a conversation Dr. Johnson we discussed one of my patients who had neck surgery for a bad disc herniation suffered as a result of a car accident, and was not getting better. He had neck surgery for a bad disc herniation he suffered as the result of a car accident. He had to modify his life just to perform the normal activities of daily living. Since he was always in chronic pain, his quality of life was poor. A group of other doctors joined the discussion and said they had similar cases. They had similar cases and agreed that if the patient does not address his METABOLIC issues with nutrition and diet, he will not get better. This was an epiphany to me. Since then looking at the metabolic issues has been effective with my patients. Of course, any successful improvement depends on whether a person will comply. It is my belief that the metabolic issues do trump everything else in terms of treatment for chronic pain conditions.

I also offer a five week weight loss program consisting of nutritional products along with caloric restriction. The nutritional products help curb the appetite naturally, so the body can burn current body fat for energy. You then have a two to three week stabilization phase where you re-set the brain to this new leaner bodyweight reducing the chances for gaining the weight back. I am constantly flabbergasted by how many weight loss commercials there are currently on television. You have the pre-packaged meals which all stay in the 1200-1600 daily caloric area. They say the glycemic index, or rate at which a food turns to sugar in your gut, is low on these foods. The truth is that, with the caloric intake this low, most people will lose weight from the calorie deprivation. However, the key is willpower. Most people are too hungry to continue with caloric restriction for long periods. In other words most people are probably eating well over 2000-2500 calories per day or more and wonder why they cannot lose weight. The nutritional value of these pre-packaged foods is nil. Their ingredients consist of all of the evils I previously explained. I will offer explain a healthy meal plan and offer dietary guidelines which I personally follow.

There are many supplements on the market. Everywhere you turn someone is selling vitamins, minerals and herbs. So where does one start? I have found through my contacts with the neurometabolic group, what I think is the best nutritional supplement company. I will go into a lot of detail later in chapter 14 because this is so important. These supplements involve what is known as a resonant frequency. This resonant frequency component relates to the energy medicine treatment I provide that I have previously mentioned.

CHAPTER TEN

Chiropractic

Most people do not realize it, but as I said in the beginning of this book, chiropractors only see about **7%** of the population. This is actually down from 10% of the population that chiropractors used to see years ago. The drug companies' advertising has been extremely effective that so many people take a variety of non-steroidal anti-inflammatories such as Advil, ibuprofen etc. Think of how many patients we chiropractors could help by just cutting back on these particular over the counter drugs. Side effects could be drastically reduced. Now if we are only seeing 7% of the population, what does that mean? Many of the total 60,000 chiropractors in the world share the same patients. Patients seem to bounce from one chiropractor to another and sometimes return to the original. I often hear patients tell me, "so and so chiropractor was busy today so I came here." Others may say the previous chiropractor hurt them or did not "get it just right" with the adjustment. In fact, many patients really treat chiropractic offices as emergency rooms and want us to be available 24 hours a day. The problem is, however, that we do not have the budget or staff to be open long hours; we are not a hospital. In fact, insurance companies classify us specialists". Look at our medical counterpart's specialists, particularly orthopedists or physiatrists-who are medical doctors specializing in physical medicine and rehabilitation. If you call them when you hurt your back, they tell you to go to the emergency room or schedule an appointment that will be at least 2-6 weeks away (although some may have 24 hour on call service). This is even true in the big offices where there may be 15 or more doctors. Think about this the next time you try to get into a chiropractor's office and are having difficulty with the schedule. There are no "chiropractic emergency room" facilities around this area.

The longer I am involved in this profession, the more I realize that I want to make a difference with those patients suffering from such chronic problems as disc problems, or stenosis (not enough room in the spinal canal) that have been with them for months or years. Many people who had surgery and are still in pain are known in the medical world as failed surgery cases.   They need a series of treatments to overcome their problem. I love to help these chronic patients who have not gotten better after seeing a list of doctors.

What is involved in the chiropractic treatment? Again, the typical patient will call my office usually with some type of back or neck pain. This can be something that just happened, acute pain, or it could be a pain that has been with them for months or years, known as a chronic pain. The first thing I do is a consultation and examination to determine the causative factors of his current condition.

Next I will formulate a treatment plan and determine which type of procedure would be best for each patient's particular condition. Influencing factors are: age, severity of symptoms, and body composition in terms of fragile or strong, etc. Next, I may tell the patient that it is standard in the industry (research has determined) that the best way to improve any condition is a two week trial treatment plan to elicit any positive response. Usually this involves three visits per week for two weeks or two visits per week for three weeks. On occasion, with serious conditions in which the patient is not sleeping and cannot perform the normal activities of daily living without extreme discomfort, I have seen a patient daily for a week.

Many patients do not understand what I am trying to accomplish. They think a chiropractor will just adjust their spine to "line it up" and that they should go to the office once in a while or when they injure themselves. Remember, I have a full service chiropractic office. Not only do I perform maintenance in which the spine is adjusted keeping everything limber, but I also treat any injuries in a prescribed number of visits as well. Since I am also certified in physical therapy among other therapies, patients can come to my office with any types of strain/sprain injuries. It is sometimes frustrating that many of the patients will only give chiropractic one or two visits and will then go to their family doctor or their orthopedic surgeon only to hear them echo my diagnosis and refer them to a physical therapist. I often find that once patients go through a series of treatments, at my office, and re-injure themselves or have a flare-up sometime later, they assume they will have to go through a three visits per week for one month treatment regimen again. With a flare-up sometimes, only one visit may get them back on track but usually it will take a few. Do not get once per month maintenance visits mixed up with a flare-up. Flare-ups, can take anywhere from 1-6 weeks to get better requiring much more treatment than just one visit.

After a diagnosis is made, the patient often asks, "What technique do you use". There are literally hundreds of chiropractic techniques. Most patients, as I have said, have never been to a chiropractor since we are only seeing 7% of the population. But for those 7%, Diversified is probably the most common technique of the chiropractic adjustment. This is performed manually. Hand contact is made to an area of the spine; the tissue slack is firmed up, and the passive range of motion is taken to end range. Next a quick impulse type force is applied by the chiropractor in an attempt to "cavitate" or open up the joint space. I must have explained the popping noise one hears during an adjustment a million times in my twenty three years of adjusting patients. The noise you hear during an adjustment is from a gas in the joint that is under pressure. This gas consisting of carbon dioxide and nitrogen is dissolved in synovial fluid which is in a capsule that surrounds the joint. When the joint space is opened, the capsule walls expand and lower the pressure so the gas comes out of the fluid and bubbles in the synovial fluid and thus makes the noise. After the adjustment, when the joint returns to normal position, the gas will redissolve in the synovial fluid and it will then make a popping noise if adjusted again. This process usually takes about twenty minutes.

Incidentally, this is the same noise you hear when you crack your knuckles. By the way, cracking your knuckles does not cause arthritis or enlarge them. For this to happen there would have to be sufficient sprain or trauma to the ligaments or soft tissues surrounding the joint. To cause any real harm or long-term damage you have to cause damage to the joint capsule for example; an overextension ligament injury by which your thumb is forced back a lot farther than it wants to go. There you have it; the knuckle cracking causing arthritis is an old wives tale.

Here are the benefits of the adjustment; but first let me mention some of the other ways of delivering an adjustment. This is where the word "technique"' comes into play. Along with asking me about the techniques I use, patients also ask me "where did you go to school?" The "technique" is referring to how you deliver the adjustment. I explained in the beginning of this book that there are "straight" and "mixer" chiropractors who only deliver an adjustment or add physical therapy to the adjustment respectively. The straight chiropractor's procedure of delivering a high velocity thrust with a certain line of drive on a patient's spine is called an adjustment. Most mixer chiropractors will refer to this "same scenario" as a manipulation. Moreover, the straight chiropractors argue that there is specificity to the adjustment that the manipulation just does not have. In other words the chiropractic manipulation is just too general; for example when one kid picks up the other while violently shaking him in order to "crack" his back.

The technique I use is based on chiropractic biophysics, which uses mirror image adjusting and manipulating the spine. I have more than 100 hours of postgraduate training with this technique. The late founder of CPB technique, Dr. Don Harrison, also a mechanical engineer and PhD in mathematics, proved the chiropractic school's techniques were flawed in their reasoning. In other words, their explanation of the system of spinal analysis was flawed. Dr. Harrison said you must look at the spine three dimensionally. Looking at two-dimensional X-rays, for example, and applying them to a three dimensional object creates distortions that may not be there. Therefore, it would only follow that one would base his method of correction on the wrong information. This is like the "fish have fins so since whales have fins they must be fish" analogy again. Dr. Harrison showed that the other technique's spinal correction rationale was also not even possible due to the anatomical way the ligaments of the spinal bones connect together. In other words, you would have to have sufficient ligament trauma for a spinal bone to move a lot, independently, the way the many of the techniques claimed. So to make a long story short, adjustment and manipulation are interchangeable and one can only be so specific due to anatomy. When I say either manipulation or adjustment, in a sentence, they refer to the same thing. Although this last statement will make many chiropractors unhappy, I think it deserves mentioning to put the adjustment/manipulation controversy in perspective. Let's look at the statistics on how safe chiropractic is compared to the medical machine's treatment. If the chiropractic adjustment needed to be extremely specific, wouldn't a lot of patients' conditions be worse due to the "humans make mistakes" aspect of the chiropractic treatment? Thus the more "generalness" of joint manipulation makes much more sense. There are a few upper cervical techniques that are very specific because they are directing a force over a very small surface resulting in minute spinal bone movements. I am not referring to these techniques.

To look at the many chiropractic techniques and describe them in detail is a book in itself. I will discuss those commonly used techniques among which "diversified", is the most popular one used by 85-90% of the chiropractors including me. The chiropractor delivers a high velocity, low amplitude thrust into a joint to restore proper motion of the joint. Chiropractic Biophysics is yet another technique I mentioned above in which the doctor uses diversified manipulation and mirror image adjustments concurrently. Flexion distraction is another popular technique where the chiropractor places his hand on the low back with the patient lying on his stomach. As the hand holds firm, the caudal section of the table where the patient's feet are, is slowly depressed downward and then slowly released upward in a deliberate, methodical, rhythmic motion in order to pump the disc space. Activator is yet another technique using a hand held instrument with a "mallet," like delivery. It is spring loaded and concentrated to a very small area. This technique is really based on a series of leg length checks, and is a softer technique in terms of force of delivery. There is also an arthrostim, very similar to the activator although it delivers multiple forces when the trigger is pulled unlike the activator, delivering a single impulse. We also have toggle recoil technique, which is what many of the first generation chiropractors used and only involves the first vertebra in the neck. There is no joint cavitation or "cracking" here and the headpiece supporting the patient will drop. There is sacro occipital technique, which involves blocks or wedges placed under the pelvis strategically. Many chiropractors included me, use a combination of the techniques mentioned above depending on the patient's situation.

There are many benefits of the adjustment/manipulation technique in the medical literature. The first one is pain relief. The scientific term of what manipulation causes is pre-synaptic inhibition of secondary afferent neurons. In other words, it blocks the pain receptor signals from the involved tissue from reaching the brain. Think of a nerve impulse, which carries a perception of pain, traveling along the body until it reaches the brain and is registered as pain. We can use a nerve/car to explain this. A nerve is the road, pain is the car, and the pain receptor in the brain is the garage door. The adjustment will close the garage door so the car cannot get in and, therefore, cannot register the perception of pain. Then we have another benefit of the endorphins being released. You may remember the "runners high" people talk about or the "second wind." This is referring to the endorphin release that makes the person less aware of his problem. This then leads to a secondary benefit of manipulation, the relaxation of trigger points or tight musculature which may have turned into a full blown "bad back episode "otherwise. Next, we have the increasing of the nutrient supply. It fact, the cartilage and structures inside the joint do not have a blood supply. This blood supply only reaches the outside of the joint; the inside of the joints depends on motion to get them the adequate nutrition. Remember the synovial fluid I previously mentioned when discussing cracking your knuckles? This joint motion disperses the nutrition around the joint in the synovial fluid. This joint movement is also required for removing the joint toxin waste that builds up in sedentary people. This is why we must keep moving at all ages. Because, of trauma or injury, we have muscle spasms that lock the joint, interrupting the joint nutrition process. Next we have improved joint proprioception giving one a better sense of joint position. When your joint is manipulated and your normal joint motion is restored, your brain learns this process so future joint movement ability is enhanced. A good example of this is when some older people must look down at their feet when they walk because they are unsure where they are located. Also, look at the wide receivers during a football game who have their hands and wrists taped. This makes their brains more aware of where their hands exactly are, thus enhancing their ability to catch the ball. So think of increased proprioception like an increase in coordinated movement. This is controlled by the cerebellum or hindbrain, as you will read shortly.

Another benefit of manipulation is reduced pressure on nerves. When a nerve adheres to any surrounding soft tissue, it can become inflamed and rigid. Then here can be pressure on the nerve or nerve tension. You can also have a bulging disc, involving the structures between spinal bones that function like shock absorbers in your car. They can also put pressure on the nerve.

These are the benefits of chiropractic manipulation that are the most widely accepted. There are many more benefits of chiropractic including somatovisceral effects that occur when an area of the spine relates to a specific organ. It is an accepted medical fact, however, that a gallbladder attack will refer pain to the tip of the right shoulder blade and an irritated lower back facet joint will refer to the groin area. Those of us who provide giving manipulations all have many anecdotal experiences of "miraculous" cases. The first chiropractic adjustment, given by B.J Palmer, resulted in a deaf janitor's hearing being restored due to the adjustment of a vertebra in his thoracic spine. There also benefits of adjustments strengthening the immune system after which those patients do not get a cold or the flu as often. Adjustment may also lower blood pressure is yet another benefit. There are some case studies on both of these last two benefits, but the mechanism is not fully understood.

To answer the question of "is chiropractic effective," we have to look at some actual studies undertaken. I will offer some studies which provide scientific legitimacy for chiropractic because; the medical profession and the drug companies have broadcasted repeatedly that it is so unscientific. When doling out a prescription the medical doctor or his assistant will say, "Try this and if it doesn't work we will try this," and so on... Does that sound scientific to you or like an exact science? How about trial and error? I already discussed that there are literally no **TOTALLY** objective studies in the drug industry.

In 1994 the Agency for Health Care Policy and Research (AHCPR) -part of the U.S Department of Health and Human Services- found in their study "Acute Low Back Problems in Adults" that spinal manipulation "is a recommended and efficacious form of initial treatment for acute low back pain in adults."

A study commissioned by the Ministries of Health in Ontario, Canada, in 1993 called, "The Effectiveness and Cost Effectiveness of Chiropractic Management of Low back pain," concluded that chiropractic management is greatly superior to medical management in terms of scientific validity, safety, cost-effectiveness and patient satisfaction. According to the study results, "there would be highly significant cost savings if more management of low back pain was transferred from physicians to chiropractors." There is also empirical evidence that patients are very satisfied with chiropractic management of low back pain and considerably less satisfied with physician management.

The College of William and Mary and the Medical College of Virginia did a study in 1992 entitled, "Mandated Health Insurance Coverage for Chiropractic Treatment: An Economic Assessment, with Implications for the Commonwealth of Virginia," showed that mandating insurance for chiropractic would not increase insurance costs, and in fact, it may even reduce them! Their study showed that chiropractic is a growing component to healthcare and that "by every test of cost and effectiveness, the general weight of evidence shows chiropractic to provide important therapeutic benefits, at economic costs." The study also states that these benefits are achieved with minimal costs or impact on health insurance.

The North American Spine Society recognizes and has included chiropractic adjustment and manipulation in its clinical procedures guide for doctors treating patients with lumbosacral spinal disorders.

The N.A.S.S. is a prestigious medical organization that publishes the monthly professional journal, "Spine." Its list of recommended procedures, including Chiropractic, appears in the October 1991 issue.

In 1992 the University of Richmond conducted a study, "A Comparison of the Costs of Chiropractors versus Alternative Medical Practitioners." This study showed that chiropractic care is a "lower cost option for prominent low back related ailments" partly because insurance coverage for chiropractic is less. This study then speculated that if chiropractic care was "insured to the extent other specialties are stipulated, it may emerge as a first option for certain medical conditions", which would then of course result in a decrease in overall cost of these conditions.

The RAND Corporation, which is a one of America's most prestigious centers for research, did a two year multi-disciplinary study in 1991 called, "The Appropriateness of Spinal Manipulation for Low back Pain," validated concluded that a trial of chiropractic should be given on "uncomplicated low back pain and for acute low back pain with minor neurological findings," which is the category where the majority of low back conditions fall. The study also recommended that the appropriate trial period for chiropractic care is four weeks instead of one to three visits, which was the previously endorsed position of most medical doctors. The RAND research panel consists of medical, chiropractic, and osteopathic doctors who are recognized experts in back pain.

In 2004 there was another study called, "Dose-response for Chiropractic Care of Chronic Low Back Pain," which was published in "Spine." They concluded that there was a "clinically important effect of the number of chiropractic treatments for chronic low back pain on pain intensity and disability at 4 weeks. Relief was substantial for patients receiving care 3 to 4 times per week for 3 weeks."

The Journal of Occupational Health found that for worker's Compensation cases, chiropractic treatment was ten times cheaper than medical care. The study was done in 1991 and titled, "Cost per Case Comparison of Back Injury Claims of Chiropractic Versus Medical Management for Conditions with Identical Diagnostic Codes." They also determined that the average worker under medical care received an average of 54.5 days of compensation whereas the injured worker under chiropractic care needed only 34.5 days. The chiropractic patients were seen three times more frequently, 12.9 vs. 4.9, but at a lower cost.

The British Medical study, "Low back pain of Mechanical Origin: Randomized Comparison and Hospital Outpatient Treatment," had its findings on the front page of the London Times. "The medical authors of the study concluded that chiropractic care should be considered for inclusion in the National Health Service." The study found that chiropractic care had better results for chronic and severe back pain versus medical care hospital outpatient management. The study also found that if chiropractic care was utilized it could save the country 290,000 sick days, 13 million pounds (about $21.19 million in US dollars) in output and 2.9 million pounds (about $4.73 million in US dollars) in social security payments.

A study done by the Department of Health Services, UCLA School of Public Health in 2004 entitled, "Comparative Analysis of Individuals With and Without Chiropractic Coverage: Patient Characteristics, Utilization, and Costs," showed how access to chiropractic could reduce overall health care expenditures through several different effects; choosing chiropractic, instead of the traditional medical model especially for spinal related conditions, by having more conservative and less invasive treatments and finally the lower health service costs associated with chiropractic.

There was a U.S. medical study performed in 1988, which was reported in the Western Journal of Medicine, called "Managing Low Back Pain Care- A comparison of the Beliefs and Behaviors of Family Physicians and Chiropractors." This study compared medical doctors and chiropractors in their attitude and approach to patients with back pain. The findings are not surprising to me. They found that MDs are not as confident with their low back treatment training and are less confident in preventing chronic back pain. They polled both the chiropractors and medical doctors on the question of doctor's poor training with lower back pain. Forty two percent of MDs agreed with only five percent of chiropractors agreeing. The next statement read, "Doctors (MD or DC) can do a lot for patients in preventing acute back pain from becoming chronic." Only 37% of the MDs agreed with this or showed confidence in their ability to treat back pain. Ninety eight percent of the chiropractors agreed to this statement.

This is a no brainer here. Wouldn't you think a medical professional who specializes in spinal conditions is going to be more confident than a professional who receives very little training in spinal related conditions? Why are the general practitioners seeing everybody and chiropractors only 7% of the population? It all comes down to money.

The last study I will discuss confirms that chiropractic is one of the few proven treatments for chronic whiplash. This study was done in 1999 entitled, "A Symptomatic Classification of Whiplash Injury and the Implications for Treatment." It was published in the Journal of Orthopedic Medicine and proved not only the superiority of chiropractic treatment in chronic whiplash patients, but also which patients respond best to chiropractic care. The conclusion was, "Our results confirm the efficacy of chiropractic with 69 out of 93 patients (74%) improving following treatment."

I must address the question, "Is chiropractic safe?" Most, if not all, of the discussions concerns the neck adjustment or manipulation possibly leading to a stroke. I am going to go over some statistics on how safe chiropractic really is. The incidence of someone suffering from a stroke following cervical adjustment or manipulation is ½ to 2 per one million treatments! Of these unfortunate individuals, one third will have mild residual damage. This number may be low because medical machine exploits chiropractic mishaps but much less frequently you hear about good outcomes. The risk from dying from a stroke following a neck adjustment is I in 4,000,000. There is about 1000 times greater a risk dying from an ulcer by gastrointestinal bleeding resulting from a prescription of NSAIDS (non-steroidal anti-inflammatories) such as Motrin. Keep the stroke risk in perspective. If a chiropractic patient drives eight or so miles to the office each way he has a statistically greater chance of being killed or seriously injured, while in transit, than from the chiropractic treatment itself.

We must also consider the possibility that in some cases the adjustment or manipulation in question, in particular stroke cases, was delivered by a medical practitioner who has far less training and experience. Furthermore, it has been determined that by the time these patients present to chiropractic offices, displaying the symptoms of a severe headache or with intense neck pain, they are already in the beginning process of undergoing strokes. A competent chiropractor carefully examines the patient looking for warning signals of an impending stroke. If any warning signals are found a prompt emergency room referral is indicated.

We have a great record of proficiency and safety in the chiropractic profession. Just look at our malpractice costs, which remain among the lowest in the entire health profession. In spite of periodic media sensationalism, the facts show that chiropractic treatments rank among the safest and most effective health care ever offered.

Let's look at the difference in the amount of hours in chiropractic and medical school. To become a chiropractor one must meet challenging educational requirements. The following lists the basic educational requirements for medical school graduates and chiropractors:

Medical Class hours		Chiropractic Class hours
508	Anatomy	520
328	Physiology	420
401	Pathology	205
325	Chemistry	300
114	Bacteriology	130
324	Diagnosis	420
112	Neurology	320
148	X-Ray	217
144	Psychiatry	65
198	Obstetrics/gynecology	65
156	Orthopedics	225
2,756	**Total Hours**	**2,887**

Other required subjects for the Doctor of Chiropractic are: adjusting, manipulation, and kinesiology. There are also 600 hours of externship qualifying the graduate for licensure in all states. In most states the chiropractor must pass a basic science exam; the same one given to medical students. The chiropractor must also pass a rigid

National and State board examination. Afterwards the state requires continuing educational seminars for annual license renewal.

Other required subjects for the Doctor of Medicine are: pharmacology, immunology, and general surgery.

GRAND TOTAL CLASS HOURS (including other Basic Subjects)

MEDICAL class hours = 4,248   CHIROPRACTIC class hours = 4,486

Note: The previous information was taken from reviewing the curriculum of twenty two medical schools and eleven chiropractic colleges. It was recently updated by the National Health Federation bulletin.

After graduation, the medical doctor needs a three year hospital residency for additional training before he can practice on his own; many doctors who specialize requires many more years. I am not trying to downplay their education. In fact they are extremely, highly educated and were among the top of their classes. I just want to emphasize that a chiropractic education consists of just as many hours minus the residency. I must also mention that what is absent from either curriculum is nutrition. All of the Formal nutritional training and certification I have is post graduate; add to these my life experiences gained from living a "health and fitness" lifestyle I have been following for the past thirty four years.

I talked above about what chiropractic is and showed studies proving its effectiveness-both clinically and in terms of cost. I also showed that we chiropractors are highly educated and trained. Now I want to discuss what kinds of conditions we see and particularly what conditions I see.

Chiropractors have a huge scope of practice and in certain rural areas in some states, where there is no medical doctor, are even allowed to deliver babies. In Pennsylvania, pap smears are in our scope of practice. I know that sounds bizarre but it is true. These practices vary from state to state. Pennsylvania also has a very liberal policy on nutrition whereas New York's scope of practice, for example, is more limited.

If we are trying to remove any stressors from the body to allow healing itself- which is the main premise of chiropractic, it makes sense that most symptoms people are suffering from are conditions chiropractors treat. We are really not treating the symptoms or the condition, however, but the person who has the symptom or condition. This is a holistic approach.

The previous studies cited all concerned how effective chiropractic care is for back and neck pain and are most of what I treat on a daily basis. Low back pain is the most common problem people present with; incredibly, statistics show that 85% of all people will have incapacitating lower back pain at some time in their lives.

Headaches are also a common condition seen by chiropractors. These are termed "tension headaches," where the pain is at the base of the neck, in the back of the head, or right behind the eyes. The tension on the upper back and trapezius muscles pulls the muscles at the back of the skull, which then due to their connections, pulls on the orbital muscles around your eyes. Many people think they are having vision problems and visit the eye doctor. Chiropractic treatment works great for this. When the range of motion is restored in the neck, nerve pressure is reduced, and the muscle spasm or tight muscles are restored to normal tension. Often the headaches seem to miraculously disappear. In addition to these tension headaches, there are also migraine headaches which I will soon discuss.

Carpal tunnel syndrome is another condition most chiropractors treat, a repetitive or cumulative trauma disorder resulting in pain, numbness and tingling in the fingers and hand. Often times there is accompanying grip strength weakness such as an inability to open jars. The culprit with carpal tunnel pain is most often the brachial muscles in the forearm. You also must keep in mind that the nerve involved in carpal tunnel syndrome, the median nerve, is formed from the nerves in your mid to lower neck. We also have to make sure that this is functioning normally. The nervous system is very complex; branches of nerve roots supply multiple structures thanks to something called the brachial plexus. For the sake of simplification, let's just say the upper back is also affected by the lower neck nerves. Therefore, I treat each one of these areas because they support the patient with carpal tunnel involvement. Sometimes we also use traction on the wrist to relieve the pressure on the carpal bones that crowd the median nerve. I also do an adjustment to these carpal bones to relieve nerve pressure and restore any lost joint motion. Over the years, I have seen many post-surgical carpal tunnel patients who usually get initial relief from surgery, but then the scar tissue grows over the excised area. Many times within a couple of years, the symptoms return because these patients did not avoid the causal repetitive motion. The main reason is that these patients must return to a job which constantly stresses the same structures. Moreover, a surgical complication causes new problems. In addition to returning, with hand tingling and pain, comes impaired motor function of the median nerve. What seems like easy task prior to surgery, like opening jars and writing, now seem impossible after surgery? Many carpal tunnel surgery patients have two or three unsuccessful surgeries after which they must go on total disability because their hands don't function properly. A Chicago surgeon told me at a conference a few years ago, that in her experience, carpal tunnel syndrome surgery is unnecessarily performed 99% of the time. She also said the motive is usually monetary.

Hip pain is another problem many people present with. Keep in mind, however, that 80% of hip pain usually has some form of lower back involvement. The joints of the lower back can also refer pain to the hip so we have to figure out exactly where the pain originates. In a hip condition, the involved muscles form knots because one muscle is overused while others are not used enough; thus we have a muscle imbalance resulting in hip pain. As a person's posture changes due to age and/or trauma, for example, certain smaller muscles begin to take over the job that global or large muscles should perform and no longer can. We all have seen those retired men, such as mail carriers, whose job involved a lot of forward flexion. After retiring, these poor men cannot even stand up straight anymore. Their bodies are doing all they can to keep the head above the shoulders to maintain a center of gravity. I must mention a soft tissue technique that is really separate from chiropractic but, since the spinal bones are held by muscles and tendons, I use it very often in conjunction with a chiropractic adjustment.

This is the trigger point technique, a soft tissue treatment in which I apply pressure to certain parts of the muscle to relax it. There is also myofascial release treatment that I often do use to break up any fascial adhesions and again restore normal tissue movement. The body has a covering over the muscle called fascia which resembles the thin transparent covering you see on chicken breast. The fascia, which should glide freely over the muscle, often contains adhesions, restricting normal muscle movement. Therefore, I will hold firm pressure on the muscle in question and have the patient move that muscle through its normal range of motion against my resistance. There is a crucial link between muscles and joints in the body. Most pain syndromes people have involving major joints in the body have some degree of trigger points and fascial restriction. **Having an alkaline pH also keeps the myofascial adhesions and trigger points to a minimum. Remember this when I talk about pH in an upcoming**

chapter. There has to be some muscular involvement along with the joint. For example, someone with hip pain who has a history of ankle sprains may also have groin pain because compensation for the weak ankle will unfortunately force the gluteal and tensor fascia lata muscles to become dominant. These large muscles, on the butt and side of your thigh, will then rotate your leg internally. This result is groin pain.

I previously mentioned that I joined the "Johnson Group" in order to provide a better service to you – the patient, from the knowledge gained from the 450 doctors in this group. **One of the main things I have learned is the way I can use more neurology and "neuro" treatments to really enhance my other treatments and get even more successful outcomes.** Now my "normal musculoskeletal (sprain/strain) chiropractic practice" has to be redefined or expanded since this additional neurology system of diagnosis and treatment has allowed me to treat more chronic conditions such as vertigo or dizziness, migraine headaches, fibromyalgia etc.

Since this is entirely new to you, let me explain how I incorporate neurology, the study of nerves, into my practice. Chiropractors look at how the brain communicates with the rest of the body through nerves. Traditional chiropractic theory is based on influencing spinal nerves by manipulating the spine in order to restore the proper communication between the brain and body. With neuro treatment, we look at other areas of the body we can treat to improve this communication. Thus, -if we alter the way we analyze this communication, we can use many different forms of treatment to remedy any problems. What is really going on, especially with chronic patients, is a brain imbalance in which one side of the brain is overactive and the other side is underactive; this will result in a decrease in the firing rate of impulses going to the structures that the underactive brain corresponds to.

This is a good time to mention the somatotopic map and a drawing called the Cortical Homunculus, a drawing of the human body with its proportions corresponding to the amount of area the brain designates to it. In other words for both motor (where the brain controls movement of the body) and sensory (tells your brain what you feel) input, a large amount of the brain is designated to the hands, feet, face, and especially the lips and tongue. So picture a man with a large face, huge hands, feet, lips, and a tongue. Due to the small amount of somatotopic representation in the brain designated to the lower back, it is no wonder why 85% of the population will suffer from incapacitating lower back pain at some point in their life.

The neurology I learned from Dr. Johnson, a Carrick trained board certified neurologist, is based on his first book *"What Do You Do When the Medications Don't Work?"*, in which he explains how the left (front) brain controls the right side of your body and the right brain controls the left side of your body. Coordinated movement and balance, so you do not fall over, are controlled by the part of your brain called the cerebellum. This is your hind brain or rear brain and it also controls termination of eye movement so the eyes do not overshoot when looking left or right. Stimulation to your right cerebellum will fire impulses in your left cortex or front brain; stimulation to your left cerebellum will fire impulses to your right front brain.

I do a neurological exam on patients to check the cranial nerves by some examples including the following: checking the sense of smell, checking certain eye movements and whether the pupil constricts to light, and checking to see if the tongue is straight when stuck out. There are also cerebellar tests such as a tandem walk and a finger-to-nose test. I will describe the cerebellum or hindbrain a little more in detail so that you can clearly understand about what is involved with many of these chronic pain problem cases. The cerebellum is divided into three parts. The top part or upper brain stem is known as the mesencephalon. The middle brain stem is the pons, and the lower region is called the medulla. Anything dealing with the lower two areas is usually referred to as the ponto- medullary region. In fact, we find that most chronic pain patients suffering from migraines, fibromyalgia, dizziness, etc. all have an increased firing of the upper brainstem or mesencephalon. The impulses to the cortex or front brain are supposed to fire to the lower brainstem or the pont- medullary region which should slow down or inhibit this upper brain stem. Thus, if the lower brainstem area does not limit the upper brain stem area, the upper brain stem area will fire at a very high rate. Here are some of the symptoms of a high firing mesencephalon or upper brain stem which many chronic pain patients exhibit: increased heart rate or tachycardia, light sensitivity, sleeplessness, increased sweating, chronic fatigue, and even a hard time emptying the bladder. A migraine patient's sensitivity to light is because his pupils will not constrict due to a decreased firing of the third cranial nerve. Guess where this third cranial nerve is located? It is in the mesencephalon or upper brain stem. The high firing mesencephalon also inhibits a person's ability to go to the bathroom. If the lower brain stem does not slow it down, the patient will not be able to void the bladder as easily and may be subject to frequent urinary tract infections. Blood pressure is also affected by a high firing mesencephalon. Like the process with emptying the bladder, the lower brain is supposed to slow the impulses of the upper brain to regulate blood pressure. Otherwise these stressed out chronic disease patients suffer from high blood pressure. Thus if one side is higher than the other, it indicates the side of decreased brain frequency of firing. I find this subject really fascinating and of crucial importance.

I want to explain some of the treatments I do when I find a brain imbalance. The first one is the adjustment/manipulation. I had never heard of an adjustment used to affect brain balance until I learned it from Dr. Johnson who explains the rationale behind the way the adjustment works on the cerebellar side. For instance, you can assess the cerebellum with tests similar to those during a police sobriety check; when a policeman makes a suspect do a finger to nose test or a tandem walk he is really assessing cerebellar function. The form of treatment I will use is a spinal adjustment to one side of the body only; the side of cerebellar findings. This is known as "unilateral adjusting'". By a feed forward mechanism, due to the anatomy of the spinal cord tracts, the adjustment will then affect the opposite side of the body, thus increasing the firing rate of impulses to the decreased brain side. If I want a lower frequency, I will use a hand held adjustment; for a higher frequency, I will use a manual/hand adjustment. I often find that these chronic pain sufferers cannot stand too much in the way of stimulus or they actually may get EMC'd, which means I exceeded their metabolic capacity to process the stimulus delivered. With these chronic suffering patients, I proceed slow and easy. Other treatment includes adjusting the extremities: foot, toes, knee, ankle, elbow, wrist, or fingers to affect the opposite side of the brain. There is also auditory stimulation where I have the patient listen to Mozart. A Mozart sonata in a major key stimulates the opposite brain. Therefore, I would have patients only listen to it in one ear. There are also nature sounds that affect the opposite brain.

Here are some home treatments I learned from Dr. Johnson which are quite easy to incorporate and powerful in what they accomplish brain/body balance. Eye exercises, a slow tracking of an object to one side followed by a sudden return back to where you started will stimulate the front brain on one side and the back brain on the other. I might have patients due word searches at home to activate the left brain and mazes that will activate the right brain. Looking at familiar faces will activate the left brain and unfamiliar faces will activate the right brain. Additionally, I can use TENS (Trans Electrical Nerve Stimulation) at a sub threshold level where the patient cannot feel it. This will decrease pain and stimulate the function of the opposite brain. There is also vibration therapy which activates the back part of the spinal cord stimulating the position receptors in the rear brain and then those in the joints, telling the body where it is in space. I previously spoke about these proprioceptors when discussing the athletes taping their wrists for better performance. There are also warm water calorics which I will explain shortly. Another therapy called a UBE (upper body ergometer), a two pedal device that one "rides "with your arms stimulating the same side cerebellum and opposite front brain. Many times I will give "spin therapy" as an exercise to be performed at home that will stimulate the endolymph in the ear canals like the action of the warm water caloric treatment. Spinning to the right stimulates the right hindbrain. Oxygen is another treatment all chronic pain sufferers should utilize. Humans only breathe in 14% pure oxygen. Since most chronic pain patients do not have a high enough oxygen perfusion I use 90% pure concentrators. Most chronic pain patients do not have a high enough oxygen perfusion rate getting the oxygen to the tissues. What is the most oxygen dependent tissue in the body? The cerebellum or hindbrain is. The brain needs two things to survive: Fuel and activation. The oxygen provides the activation and what we eat supplies the fuel when it is turned into glucose. Olfactory stimulation (smell therapy) can be used to stimulate the brain on the same side. There is a squeezable hand ball which stimulates the same side cerebellum. I have patients do an exercise where they pretend to swim the backstroke for 3 minutes, 3 times per day to increase the impulses to the cerebellum.

Let's look at vertigo, or dizziness, and I will discuss some examples of how to evaluate and treat a dizziness complaint. This is a severe this problem is in our country; forty percent of adults over 40 years of age will succumb to a dizziness disorder at some time in their lives. Falls due to balance problems account for 50% of elderly deaths. Over 90 million Americans have experienced a bout with dizziness or a balance problem.

With concentric vertigo, the patient feels as if the room is spinning around him; in egocentric vertigo he feels as if he is flying around the room. Medical doctors will often diagnose the dizziness as an inner ear disturbance, which leads to a diagnosis of BPPV (benign paroxysmal positional vertigo). Normally the body maintains its balance with the help of tubes called semicircular canals. Sometimes calcium crystals or "canalith" can float into the fluid in these canals causing BPPV. Usually the treatment of choice is canalith repositioning, or Epply's Maneuver, performed to rearrange these crystals out of the canal fluid. I can perform this maneuver in the office if necessary. When a patient tells me he has chronic dizziness and has seen a medical doctor for it, I assume he has been prescribed the drug Meclizine. The fact that he is still complaining of it means that either the drug was not indicated or it was ineffective. In some instances, the Canalith repositioning will take care of the patient and if he does the exercises periodically he will be fine. However, if the problem is more complicated than that usually a decrease rate of firing on one side of the brain versus the other is the cause.

Let's look at a recent patient, in his early fifties, presenting to my office with back pain. During his course of treatment, I also found he suffered from chronic dizziness and never saw a medical doctor, since "It would come and go" he said. A neurological exam discovered that his right cerebellum and left cortex (front brain) were weak and not firing as strongly as his left cerebellum and right cortex. He said some other practitioner attempted to perform the canalith repositioning but was unsuccessful. When he lay on his back, the patient's dizziness was so magnified he had to get up. I did a unilateral (one sided) chiropractic adjustment with the patient seated to stimulate the right side- the affected cerebellar side. This affected the opposite frontal cortex or brain. I also decided to give him a warm water caloric in his right ear with a syringe 60 ml of distilled water at 105 degrees. The head was tilted forward and to the opposite direction in this case to the left, accounting for the angle of the ear canal. The water ran in and out of the ear concurrently. No water remained in the ear. There is a gel called endolymph in the semicircular ear canals These semicircular canals also contain hair cells called stereocillia and kinocillia. The warm water turned the gel like endolymph, in my patient's ear, to a more of a watery consistency. This action stimulated these hair cells allowing the vestibular nerve to then fire back to the cerebellum thus increasing its rate of firing. This patient received immediate relief and was able to lie down on his back without getting dizzy. Since nerve impulses travel extremely fast, we often get immediate results with this procedure. This was the first time the patient ever had relief during an episode of dizziness and agreed to perform the home eye exercises I prescribed keeping the stimulation to the right cerebellum and left cortex.

In most chronic diseases and migraine headache cases, I almost invariably see some imbalance between the left and right brain firing; one side is over firing while the other is under firing. As with the dizziness treatments, I have different treatment options to increase the firing of one side of the brain while slowing down the other to attain proper balance. As a result many of my chronic conditions patients, who have "tried everything", got better.

CHAPTER ELEVEN

More Therapies Offered

I now discuss the modalities or therapies I use every day. Some are used concurrently with adjustment/manipulation and some are used independently not only the musculoskeletal conditions or back and neck pain, ankle, knee, wrist sprains etc. I may also use these with chronic conditions like fibromyalgia, migraine headaches, chronic fatigue syndrome, and many others.

Next I will explain each modality, giving examples of how and why I use them. **Therapeutic ultrasound** is a therapy everybody confuses with the diagnostic ultrasound used on women to view a growing fetus. Deeply penetrating therapeutic ultrasound on the other hand works by vibrating a crystal in the sound head of the machine which produces heat, creating blood flow to the involved tissues to enhance healing. It also warms up the tissues for the traction therapy discussed in the next chapter because I use it every traction patient. Although this is excellent, for all sprains and strains, it cannot be done over a boney prominence.

Electro therapy increases the blood flow to the involved tissues enhance healing, and reduce any muscle spasm breaking the pain/spasm cycle that many patients suffer after an injury like an irritating sprain/strain. Among the many different kinds of electrotherapy, the TENS current is used by many patients who have home. This acronym stands for transcutaneous electrical nerve stimulation. Another electrotherapy treatment is interferential current by which two fast frequencies cross resulting in a medium frequency that is very comfortable to the patient. There is also hi-volt galvanic, very good for inflammation and muscle spasm. Electrotherapy is also part of the protocol I use with traction/decompression to help with the muscle spasms. As previously discussed, TENS can also be used to balance the low firing brain with the other over firing side. We apply it at a sub threshold level opposite hemisphere and the same side cerebellum.

Intersegmental traction is another of my therapies that some of my patient's call the "roller table". A roller in this table gently separates each vertebra on its way up and down over your spine while you relax on your back. This also activates the proprioception.

Whole body vibration is another modality that is great for total body health. The patient simply stands on a vibrating platform and holds on. Anyone can exercise on this if your balance is good. The vibration plate works by generating vibrations in the plate base, and the vibrating force is then transferred directly through the entire body causing all the muscles to contract and relax. The lower speed vibration helps to refresh and relax the body, whereas the high speed vibration creates intense and rapid muscle contractions. This vibration plate is a great machine for those of you who spend most of the day sitting at home or in the office. Research has shown that 10 minutes on a vibe plate is equal to 60 minutes of regular exercise!

Benefits:

- Improves and increases your muscle strength, body shape, tone and posture.
- Helps to burn unwanted fat, combat cellulite, tighten your skin and improves your body's natural collagen levels.
- Improves joint movement and increases flexibility.
- The massaging motion eases aches and pains (low speeds).
- Reduces tiredness, stress and reduces your back, muscle and joint pain.
- Increase metabolism, helping to burn fat and raise energy levels while improving digestion.

- Improves your blood circulation and lymphatic drainage which improves joints, cartilage, decreases blood pressure and cortisol levels.
- Quick recovery from joint, muscle and ligament injuries.
- Strengthens bones and fights osteoporosis.
- Strengthens the pelvic floor and improves continence.
- Improves balance, coordination and core stability.
- Increases energy levels and improves overall fitness.

Decompression and ATM (applied therapeutic motion) – Having had a lot of postgraduate training in a variety of treatment techniques that I use daily treating a variety of conditions, such as neck and back sprain/strain, carpal tunnel, and various types of headaches, I became also interested in treating disc injury cases. In 2001, I bought a table which would allow me to treat these disc cases using decompression. I also became certified in spinal decompression that same year. In chiropractic there has been a paradigm shift over the last fifteen years from the conservative treatment of lower back disorders most notably disc cases. I love the quote by Abraham Maslow that holds so true. He said, "When all you have is a hammer, everything looks like a nail." This echoes how many doctors do one form of treatment and try to fit everybody into that form. The results, from this sole means of treatment are usually not that good. Before the decompression became available, we had limited options how to treat these patients; electrotherapy, adjustment/manipulation, ultrasound, and rehab or active exercise. Today, over 15% of chiropractors use decompression therapy. Decompression is an accessory motion the patient cannot do on his own. Yes, you can hang from an inversion table and get about 3-4mm of separation at the lowest lumbar vertebra, but it is unable to provide the necessary pull/relax cycle. The spinal cord does not like static traction the way it does intermittent traction therefore the decompression is the means to deliver this intermittent traction.

Many people are unfamiliar with what a disc is; I will provide a quick explanation of the disc and its function. (The word disc can be spelled either disc or disk both is correct.) The disc is in between the vertebra. There are twenty four vertebra and twenty three discs in the spine. The discs normally function as a buffer for the vertebra above and below them. They hold water and actually protect the vertebra above and below them which also allows for bending and movement. A non-degenerated disc is very strong and will not fail before the bone will. But once it is degenerated due to age, poor posture, physical abuse, genetics etc., it will be exponentially weaker. Comprised of a center or nucleus, composed of 88% water, it is surrounded by a ligament called the annulus fibrosis, patterned in concentric circles running parallel to each other. Normally water flows in and out of the disc through tiny pores. Whenever a person sits or stands, weight bearing on the spine makes the spine loaded squeezing the water out of the disc. On the other hand, when someone is lying down, the disc allows water to come back in. This is why you are up to an inch taller in the morning. As you age, the amount of water which leaves the spine throughout the day is greater than the water that goes back in. This is one reason why we shrink as we age. Unlike our muscles and organs, these discs have no direct blood supply. This means that for the discs to receive the necessary nutrition and for waste products to be carried away, they have to rely on mechanical means or movement and the flow of water. In the degenerated disc the border between the center of the disc or gel to the ligament or annulus is lessened. I tell patients that the discs in the back and neck are really like a jelly donut. When the gel-like center starts to push out to the side in a broad fashion you get a bulge. Furthermore, if the center pushes out in a more focused fashion or if even broken through, it becomes a herniation. Consequently, the ligament or annulus tears and gets fissures in it. This heals with scar tissue which is a grade three collagen. It is inferior in strength and is much less flexible than the original type 4 collagen that it replaces. Therefore, once you injure the disc it is always more predisposed to give you future problems. And when you reach the mid-sixties, a lot of the pressure that gives the disc strength is gone, leaving a person very weak and more prone to any compressive load type injury. The degenerated disc has very little or no water in it. Of course any patients at this stage are harder to treat since it is hard to decompress a disc that has no pressure and is already in negative nitrogen balance, a "decompressed state". The only relief these patients get is during the traction. Their pain returns immediately afterwards. This is where the K-laser comes in. I will talk about it shortly.

Unfortunately, some chiropractors who own decompression tables do not fully know how to use them. Many place the patient in the wrong position so that the patient is in agony just lying on the table before the stretching on the machine begins. Obviously, this will be a terrible outcome; the patient must be comfortable on the table for the treatment to work. Often some chiropractors pull the patient with entirely too much weight. This is a very subtle treatment and it is not necessary to use large amount of weight to be highly effective. Many clinics using this type of treatment have the chiropractic assistants, before the treatment begins, deciding these crucial matters of patient position and weight. They pretty much just "wing it" and hope for the best. This improper use of the treatment is why the profession offers the certification course. From such a course, I learned a great deal; it re-enforced what I had learned from years of study.

When evaluating a patient for traction/decompression, the chiropractor uses categorizing, in which he determines what type of pain syndrome the patient presents and if he is indeed a candidate for decompression. In this section I am talking about a disc problem. But the patient could also have a motion or movement disorder that I will discuss next, or the patient could have a combination of a disc problem and a motion disorder. I must stress that a patient needs to be categorized so the treatment outcome is favorable. Let's look at a lower back disc patient. I also treat many neck disc problems. Once I realize that the person has a disc problem, I must decide how to position him on the traction/decompression, and also decide what level of force to use. I must mention here that the word "decompression" is simply the effect of traction. When the disc pressure is reduced, during long axis traction, it allows the disc to heal. Research has discovered this decompression tends to happen with about 50 pounds of force on the lower back disc. When the patient is positioned on the table and the traction device is turned on, a tug or pulling feeling will occurs where the belt is fastened to your hips. This traction reduces the hydrostatic pressure in the disc below that of the osmotic pressure around it, allowing the fluid to diffuse into the disc. Importantly, nutrients will also diffuse into the disc space once the pressure of the disc is lower than the surrounding pressure. This treatment is so very relaxing that many of the patients will fall asleep because this is most comfortable they have been in a while. Another great therapy to use in conjunction with the decompression/traction is oxygen therapy. As previously stated, the brain and nervous system need two things: Oxygen and glucose. Dr. Mike Johnson shared with us his success stories behind using the oxygen while the patient is getting stretched with the decompression. So about two years ago, I started using the oxygen concentrators with traction on some patients and the results were even more enhanced. I have severe disc patients tell me that their cardiologists check their oxygen levels every day, and they are always within normal levels. I tell them that the brain and spinal cord *are much more sensitive to oxygen deprivation* than the rest of the body.

The motion disorder occurs when you have small intrinsic muscles, for example, the small muscles in the spine began to act like large global muscles such as the hamstrings or gluteal muscles as I earlier explained. Due to altered postures over the years from bad ergonomics at work, poor sleeping posture, traumatic injury, etc., the body adapts using any means to keep the head centered over the pubic bone. However, other parts of the spine may not be balanced. Remember what I said about the cerebellum or hindbrain controlling balance and coordinated movment? Dr. Johnson's recommendations on one of his teaching DVDs really resonated with me. He said, "When you think about those people with scoliosis, which is a deviation of the spine from midline, they should all have their brains checked for a cerebellar imbalance." This makes great sense because these people are the same ones who have always been uncoordinated and claim to always have motion sickness.

Someone who has an altered posture will eventually developed sprains and strains on the spine; actually structure does dictate function. For example, a car running on one donut tire will not run the same as when all four tires are the normal size right? When a patient with a motion disorder bends over, he is firing the wrong muscles in the wrong sequence. I have a device called ATM (applied therapeutic motion) which stabilizes a weak area enabling a new pattern of muscle firing and sequence can occur. A motion disorder is usually accompanied by a lot of pain.

Let's return to my disc patient who I find has a disc problem combined with a motion disorder; he is going to need both the traction/decompression and the ATM forms of treatment to recover. Once, I overheard my wife tell a patient that the ATM (applied therapeutic motion) machine is like an "ATM" (auto-teller machine at the bank) but it does not give you any money. Before I had the ATM, many patients would be unable to get off the traction table and often would leave feeling worse than when they came. A typical example is the disc patient who cannot bend backwards at all but can bend forward with some pain. After the traction, the patient's extension (bending back) is greatly improved, but his forward bending is a little worse. The reason is that the traction helped the disc component but irritated the motion disorder component by pulling the core. I take these patients to the ATM unit and simulate, with my hands, pressure on his hips while rocking their pelvis one way or the other and simultaneously having him bend forward to see if it takes his pain away. If this simulation is successful, I then strap the ATM belts on them and tighten them to secure the weak area. This stabilizes the weakness that is preventing them from bending pain-free. I will then have the patient try to flex or bend forward against resistance for a few isometric contractions, which they hold for three seconds. When I take any out of the ATM, almost all, in fact, 99% of them can bend further and with significantly less pain than before the treatment. This is a neurological treatment by which the brain memorizes the sequence needed to contract certain muscles allowing the bending motion to occur without pain. Thus, the treatment may seem simple and mechanical, but the mechanism of how it works is very complex. When a patient says, "It hurts when I move this way," the use of the ATM machine is indicated, also for a hip, shoulder, or neck, and not only the lower back. It can also be used as a neurological treatment for someone having a cerebellar imbalance.

Ever since I started seeing disc cases, I have had excellent results with many patients who did not want surgery or those who were not surgery cases according to their surgeon. I have even had good results with many failed low back surgery cases. Patient's with disc problems will come in and say, "I have a herniated or bulging disc." Having gone the medical route; x-rays, MRI, and CAT scan, they may even have been through one or two courses of physical therapy with no successful results. Combining the traction and ATM has really helped get even many of the toughest cases better faster.

Massage – Another treatment in an inclusive chiropractic office is therapeutic massage, performed as far back as 2700 BC for pain relief, fever and chills, and even complete paralysis. Hippocrates in the 5th century BC said, "Rubbing can bind a joint that is too loose and loosen a joint that is too rigid." Julius Caesar apparently needed daily massage to treat the neuralgia or nerve pain he suffered.

Although, there are many types of massage, most westerners know mainly the Swedish one developed by doctor and poet, Per Henrik Ling, in the 1800s. It was based on his study of gymnastics and physiology and borrowed techniques from China, Greece, Rome, and Egypt. Today, massage is used on people of all ages, from babies in the intensive care unit, to the elderly in nursing homes and even those in hospices.

This office has massage therapists specializing in a number of massage types to meet a variety of patient's needs: acupressure, Tai yoga, deep tissue, lymphatic, oncology, prenatal, Mu-Xing, hot Stone, Swedish, and sport's to name several. Our experienced therapists will customize a massage to meet an individual's needs. I will describe some of these.

Swedish massage consists of long strokes along the paraspinal muscles, targeting knots in the muscle and adhesions that prevent the tissues from moving smoothly. This is very relaxing. *Deep tissue massage* is very similar to the Swedish massage except the therapist is targeting the deepest layers of the muscle, tendons and fascia- or the protective covering over the muscles. *Lymphatic massage* concentrates on the lymph system which many people are unaware of. The blood vessels bring oxygen to the tissue and the lymph system then removes toxins, waste products and excess fluids from the spaces between the cells and filters them. Normally when the lymph system is working properly, a person has a stronger defense against illness but when blocked or sluggish after an illness or surgery, for example, he could be swelling, fatigued and more susceptible to colds and the flu. In *acupressure massage* the massage practitioner uses fingers instead of needles to apply strong pressure on acupuncture points. This is based on the meridian system which I described earlier. Acupressure increases circulation and reduces tension and pain. *Tai yoga massage* does not require use any oils and is usually performed with the patient lying on the floor. In this system of massage and assisted stretching developed in Thailand, the practitioner leans on the patient's body using his hands and usually straight forearms to apply rhythmic pressure. This type of massage is aimed at influencing the "Sen" lines on the body which are somewhat similar to the meridians.   There is also an energy technique massage, *sports massage*, used to focus on the areas that are overused from repetition or aggressive movements by elite athletes or weekend warriors, for example. It also targets the musculo-tendonous junction that will increase blood flow to the areas thus preventing the buildup of excessive scar tissue. It can also increase range of motion and has been shown to decrease muscle soreness felt either before or after exercise. Some people visit the office strictly for massage; many others receive the laser, chiropractic care, therapies and massage.

<u>CHAPTER TWELVE</u>

The K-Laser: A Stand Alone Treatment

Although Albert Einstein developed laser theory in 1916, he did not invent the laser but his photoelectric theory laid the groundwork. He was the first to discover that "stimulated emissions of radiation" can occur. This insight was the basis for the therapeutic laser. The word Laser is really an acronym for L- light, A-amplification, of S-stimulated E-emissions of R-radiation. Finding the right kind of atoms and using reflecting mirrors to help the stimulated emissions along was all that was needed to invent it.

After the first working laser was invented by Theodore Maiman it was unsuccessful because it was too underpowered and could not disperse the heat it created and reach therapeutic effects.

In 1968 a German physicist Endre Mester, known as "The father of low level laser therapy" tried to cure cancer in rats and failed but found the laser healed the incision wounds quickly. Thus the incredible healing capability of the laser was revealed. Scientists worked diligently in the next few years and found a way to get more power along with more heat dispersion and less heat build-up so that the laser was more effective and therapeutically practical. Lasers were used for over forty years in other countries but are relatively new in the United States, approved only in 2002. The class IV laser received FDA clearance here in 2003 but had been used in Europe for over ten years prior.

The class of the laser is determined by its wattage. The common laser pointer used in a presentation or a laser scope on a rifle is a class IIIA and has 1.5 mill watts of power. From 5-500 mill watts is a class IIIB which can cause eye injury if shined directly into the eye but really does not have enough power to have a therapeutic effect unless the treatment time is really extended. Power equals watts multiplied by seconds. So if you do not have the watts you have to increase the time. The class IV laser, with greater than 500 mill watts and no upper limit can be hazardous to the eyes and skin. Today most therapeutic lasers are class IV and range in power anywhere between 8 and 15 watts. My own K-laser is at the top of this range with 15 watts of power.

When people hear the word laser, many times they think of a surgical one whose purpose is to destroy tissue through excess heating and also seals or cauterizes blood vessels to limit blood loss during surgery.

In contrast, the therapeutic laser works through cells in our skin called chromophores, located in the powerhouse of the cell called the mitochondria. In the mitochondrial membranes, these chromophores absorb light and produce ATP, or the fuel of the human body, the way gas is the fuel for your car. This process is called photobiomodulation and leads to accelerated healing of tissue, pain reduction, and inflammation reduction- all simultaneously. This K-laser treats the cause of the tissue injury, not just the symptoms, and can be used immediately after an injury.

I will get a bit technical for all of you left brained Engineer/analytical types. The K-laser CUBE 4 has four treatment beams operating simultaneously measured in nanometers; the distance of light designated between successive points on the light wave. There is a visible red beam at 660 nm (nanometers) which we can see and then three infrared wavelengths at 800, 905, and 970 nm which are invisible to the naked eye. The wavelength determines therapeutic penetration of the laser. The three elements of our body which absorb more laser energy than the rest are water, melanin, (pigment in our skin determining skin darkness) and hemoglobin, (an oxygen carrying protein pigment in the blood) thus each having different absorption patterns.

Remember, the goal of therapeutic laser is to penetrate deep into the tissues to enhance and repair the regeneration process. It does this by targeting three chromophores or enzymes: cytochrome c oxidase, oxygenated hemoglobin, and water. With its four simultaneous wavelengths during treatment, the K-laser CUBE 4 delivers a wavelength of treatment radiation that lies at the peak of each of these chromophores. The 905 nm wavelength is the peak of hemoglobin's absorption making more oxygen enriched fuel for the cells to carry out their natural healing processes. Water absorbs very well at 970 nm allowing oxygen to enter the cells and waste products to be carried away resulting in an increased circulation. The melanin in our skin absorbs the 660 nm wave very well and since light can inhibit bacteria this is great for superficial wound healing. Thus it is the 800 nm wavelength that targets the cytochrome c oxidase or the end of the respiratory transport chain. This is the chromophore that determines how fast the cell converts oxygen into ATP. There is an incredible short video on our website, www.gildeachiropractic.com, which shows this process and really illustrates it well. Usually, the body will do this task at its own pace, cycling between a reduced and oxidized state. When it absorbs a photon of light from the laser, however, this process becomes accelerated 300-900% faster resulting in more ATP. What does this mean? The body will then heal 300-900% faster than it would on its own if no laser photons are absorbed. In this regard, the K-laser CUBE SERIES is the most efficient laser available targeting the body's natural healing process.

There are many who contend that there is no need for such a powerful laser to stimulate healing. To address this we must look at energy itself and how it works. For therapeutic effects of energy to be realized, the laser's energy must not only penetrate deep enough to reach the target tissues, but it must have enough energy left over to stimulate the physiological effect of promoting healing. Thus, when there is an injury and it has affected the body at different depths, various wavelengths are ideal. Some lasers are ineffective due to an inappropriate wavelength or too low a dosage. One thing to remember is that only 20-40% of the light is absorbed by the deeper target area meaning over 50% is absorbed by water and tissue below the skin.

K-LASER CUBE 4 also offers pulse frequency, a method using a 50% duty cycle in which the laser light will pulsate on and off. It will be "on" half the time and "off" the other half. This pulse frequency can vary anywhere between 2 to 20,000 Hertz. How is that for blinking fast? This enables the laser to get a lot more power to the tissues because the immense amount of heat produced will be dissipated sufficiently so that the patient can tolerate the laser.

Daniel Knapp DC, a chiropractor and trainer for K-laser USA, also a University of Miami School of Medicine Complimentary and Integrative Department laser therapy consultant, had an interesting paper in the January-February issue of the JACA (Journal of the American Chiropractic Association). He presented Class IV laser therapy as a potential intervention strategy in the treatment of resistant chronic lower back and leg pain complicated by spinal stenosis, a narrowing of the canal in the spinal column. His case study was a 77 year old female who underwent bilateral total knee replacement and total hip replacements. She presented using a walker and was in obvious discomfort. On a scale of one to ten with ten being the worst, she reported pain levels of 3 to 10, citing sharper pain across the lower back, butt, and hips. Her onset of pain was right after the hip replacement 9 months prior. Since that time she had five epidural steroid injections which did not afford her any significant relief. She did get some small relief from Oxycodone. This was complicated by a congenital disorder known as Spondyloslisthesis in which the bone above moved out in front of the vertebra below it. In this case L4 was out in front of L5. This was only a grade one so the bone above could only be 25% or less forward on the bone below. She also had an MRI confirmed L5-S1 disc protrusion hitting the thecal sac, which covers the spinal cord, and right S1 nerve root establishing multiple pain generators. In other words, this lady was a ness and a very complicated case due to her surgeries and congenital problem.

The medical profession's gold standard treatment for this case would be lower back decompressive surgery. Reviewing the medical literature shows limited studies on chiropractic care for chronic low back complicated by stenosis. The researchers had to admit, however, there were some potential benefits.

There are also limited studies on laser therapy with lower back pain. There were two papers; however, that showed laser and exercise were more effective than exercise alone. A Cochran study, in 2008, on low level laser therapy concluded that there was insufficient data to draw a conclusion.

Now let's go back to the 77 year old patient. When the treatment began, the K-LASER was the only method of treatment, a 10 watt class IV laser. She received 11 treatments over a 9 week period. Manipulation therapy was added on the fourth visit but was found to irritate her condition; it was stopped immediately. These treatments resolved her left sided pain and reduced the pain scale on the right by 50%. There was no other treatment intervention employed. Progressive reduction in pain enabled her to be more physically active which increased her range of motion and added activities of daily living that she could not previously have done due to her pain level.

The author concludes that the class IV K-laser may be a treatment option in these chronic "multi-factorial" low back pain patients because it will possibly allow them to return to normal activities of daily living sooner. There are over 2500 published studies involving laser therapy with over 100 double blind studies published.

There are also very brief videos on YouTube showing the K-laser being used and endorsed by the head trainers of the New York Yankees. Steve Donohue, their assistant athletic director of thirty years said athletes "line up for it" in the locker room. They also said of the K-laser: "I think we have gotten more rapid recoveries" and "guys are returning to the field sooner." Paul Sporting, head trainer of the Cincinnati Bengals said, "Players that have chronic lower back soreness found the only thing that gave them true relief on a consistent basis was the K-laser."

Some people might ask, what do these sports anecdotes have to do with ordinary people? On my K-laser forum, doctors from around the country discuss their cases in a similar way to the neurometabolic forum I belong to. Every problem from toe nail fungus to shingles is avidly discussed and information exchanged on-line. It is difficult to find the right protocol for some of these non-musculoskeletal problems requiring great skill, experience, and availability of other opinions. Remember the laser heals by increased blood flow/waste product removal and reduced inflammation. Thus the list of things that can be treated is almost endless. One could claim there is probably an 85% success rate overall, making this one of the most effective natural non-invasive treatments available.

In my office, I mostly treating patients for musculoskeletal disorders including the following: back pain, disc problems with radiculopathy or shooting pains down the arm or leg depending on whether a cervical or neck disc or a lumbar or lower back disc, hip and knee problems- including knee and hip replacement patients, carpal tunnel syndrome- including those who had surgery, foot and ankle problems, jaw pain, and headaches. I would say that almost everybody I ever treated with the K-Laser noticed some improvement with many of these conditions.

There are also some contraindications for laser use. laser Moreover, there are some things a laser should not be used: over growth plates or skull sutures in infants, a pacemaker or other electrical devices, to patients who had a recent cortisone injection within the past week, over hemorrhage, over tattoos- they will heat up too fast-, multiple sclerosis patients as they may heat up too fast, and any area of decreased sensory perception or numbness.

Remarkably, however, and unbeknownst to most, the K -laser therapy can be safely applied over metal implants whether they are knee or hip replacements, rods in the back or neck- or any other metal implants for that matter. The skin and tissue absorbs the heat from the laser. There is NO HEATING of the metal. Patients with joint replacements are often in chronic pain due to the altered threshold of their pain fibers from which the laser can usually give substantial pain relief.

Most people feel much better the next day. Some people may notice mild pain shortly after or the day after treatment. This only means the technique might have been too strong. The next day they will usually feel improvement. Older patients sometimes cannot tolerate as much power, thus we have to accommodate by using less.

The protocol with the K-laser is different if a patient's condition is acute which means it happened within the last two weeks. This patient needs a frequent dose with less power or intensity for a period of three visits per week for two weeks or 6 visits. The tensile strength of the injured tissues should be healed at this point. For the problem of a sub-acute condition happening within the past four weeks, a patient's treatment schedule should be two visits per week for three weeks or 6 visits. With chronic pain and overuse injuries, a patient will at least need 15 or so visits. The ideal treatment schedule for chronic disc problems is three visits per week for one week and two visits per week for maybe five weeks, and then one visit per week for a couple of weeks. Many chronic patients do not see any relief after 5 or 6 visits. Remember, chronic condition need more time to heal. The injured or affected area, devoid of a normal blood supply is now deteriorating. Thus, we need a higher laser dose to jump start the healing. This will cause angiogenesis, formation of new blood vessels, to carry oxygen rich blood to the affected area, and force the injured cells, which are usually dormant to metabolize again. Of course when dealing with a chronic patient the treatment plan is based on results and then modified accordingly.

This laser treatment is so effective but unfortunately very underutilized today. I want to end this section by including additional benefits of this laser therapy. First is accelerated tissue repair and cell growth. The laser light increases the energy of the cell so it can exchange nutrients and waste in and out of the cell faster. For those who take supplements, the laser can enhance how the body utilizes them. Many people's bodies are loaded with toxic junk from our environment, which can also be removed from the cell easier using the laser light. As a result, bones, ligaments, tendons, nerves and muscles heal and repair faster. Wounds heal faster. Certain types of cells called fibroblasts which stimulate new cells, are formed faster from the laser light, and these cells are the building blocks of collagen- which is used to replace old injured tissue. Laser therapy also reduces scar formation following surgery, burns, cuts and scratches, by producing more Type 1 collagen instead of Type 3 collagen, the inferior grade. Remember, scar tissue is the primary source of chronic pain. Laser light has an anti-inflammatory effect by increasing vasodilation of blood vessels allowing lymphatic drainage of swollen areas caused by inflammation and bruising. Pain relief is also a very important benefit of laser therapy because it positively affects the nerve cells which send pain signals from the affected area to the brain. This decreases nerve sensitivity. It also releases a lot of pain killing endorphins and enkephalins from your brain. The release of these chemicals is experienced in a runner's high. Improvement with nerve function is a major benefit with laser therapy. Since nerves heal very slowly after an injury and the damaged tissue can result in numbness and impaired muscles, laser therapy will speed up the process of nerve-cell reconnection to optimize muscle function. Finally, trigger points and acupressure points can be stimulated in a non-invasive manner (without needles) providing musculoskeletal pain relief.

Well there you have it. I cannot consider practicing without this invaluable K-laser Cube 4. Before any joint surgery or replacement surgery you are thinking of for your chronic condition, please consider a K-laser treatment protocol. For those people who choose surgery as their best course of action, keep in mind that the K-laser will significantly speed up your healing process when given right after surgery and return you to your "normal activities of daily life" faster.

CHAPTER THIRTEEN

The Metabolic Way to Health: Hope Science

It has been well documented in the literature that inflammation is indeed the culprit for all of these chronic diseases people are suffering from increasingly. Whether it is the mycoplasma organism, years of the S.A.D, exposure to toxic chemicals and heavy metals, tick bites, etc.... the result is the same: A cascade of inflammatory chemicals in the body, which as I have previously mentioned, resulting in auto immune reactions. And this results in- you guessed it- MORE INFLAMMTION.

In fact, as I have said before, unless you address the metabolic or nutritional aspects of patients, many of the chronic inflammatory muscle pain syndromes will not subside. In this section I will address what I recommend to my patients not only for preventative health maintenance, but also to bring them back to health when a problem arises.

First I want to discuss the two nutritional companies I use, Hope Science and Premier Research Labs. I learned about both from other doctors, Dr. Kevin Connors in particular, on the Johnson Group board I joined. Since that time, these highly recommended companies have been extremely effective with many of my patients. Remember, Dr. Conners wrote the book on cancer I mentioned in an earlier section.

Dr. Kim Vanderlinden, a naturopathic doctor, formed the company Hope Science, out of frustration with the poor quality of the current products on the market. His two flagship products IP6 and EFAC (esterified fatty acid cream) represented, what he thought were the two most important finds in the preventative health care field. Extremely concerned with the suffering of so many depressed patients, without any relief in sight, he desperately wanted to reduce their pain. When he gave he gave his EFAC cream to a severely depressed patient contemplating suicide. He saw hope return in the patient's eyes within 15 minutes. In Dr. Vanderlinden's own words, "Hope is why we have medicine. Science is a foundation for hope. Hence the name…. Hope Science." This company has world class researchers whose credentials are available on www.hopescience.com.

IP6, inositol + calcium and magnesium bound to six phosphates comes in capsule form. Sodium and iron could also be bound to phosphate but the Cal Mag IP6 is thought to be the most beneficial form. I highly recommend Dr. Vanderlinden's book co-authored with, Dr. Ivana Vucenik PhD., on this incredible supplement called *"Too good to be True? Prevention and Treatment of: Cancer, Osteoporosis, Depression, Diabetes, Heart disease and more."*

According to Dr. Vanderlinden, the rational for using Ip6 is to prevent cancer. Along with a healthy lifestyle, the author believes that this supplement is crucial. Although I am not writing this book on treating cancer, since cancer afflicts so many of us, I think it deserves mentioning that IP6 may help. For example, it normalizes the rate of cell division which has been lost. It enhances the ability of the natural killer cells which are very important in our immune system necessary to kill the 500 to 1000 cancer cells that the average adult produces on a daily basis. Stress reduces the natural killer cell's ability. Drug ads on television will often say when mentioning side effects, "if you have a depressed immune system" or "if you are on immune suppressing drugs do not take this drug." Prednisone is an example of an immune suppressing drug as it is a steroid composed of cortisol. (If you remember, cortisol is secreted by your adrenal cortex to fight off inflammation and boost immunity. When you take prednisone drug, your body does not produce its own and your immune system is compromised.)

IP6 also increases the P53 gene tumor suppressor activity. In one study it increased the amount by 17 times; these genes keep any genetically damaged or cancer cells from further division. I previously mentioned that HCL and methyl groups also increase the P53 gene. IP6 inhibits inflammation and is a potent antioxidant. Oxidative stress damages the DNA of our cells leaving them very susceptible which could mean mutation into cancerous cells. In comparison to green tea, also supposed to be a very powerful antioxidant, IP6 is much more potent. IP6 enhances cell suicide or natural programmed cell death which is needed for the normal maintenance of the body tissues- to remove dead cells and rebuild new ones. IP6 is antiangiogenic. Cancerous tumors require new blood vessels to be formed in order to expand and continue multiplying. They can have up to 30- 40 times the metabolic rate as normal cells. In several experiments IP6 inhibited new blood vessel growth. Lastly, IP6 inhibits the cancer cells from sticking to the extracellular matrix proteins thus preventing them from migrating or invading other tissues. This is extremely important after surgeries, when cancer will often spread by adhering to the tissues.

The "I' in IP6 stands for inositol and is found in all of the cells of the body and in the cell membranes. It is believed to be of highest concentration in the brain, sperm and testes. Along with its cancer preventing ability it is known for helping many other conditions such as: diabetic neuropathy-tingling in the feet and hands, neural tube defects, fatty liver, depression, obsessive compulsive disorder, brain seizures, cholesterol and triglyceride levels, and as an anti-oxidant against premature aging. Inositol is considered to be part of the B complex of vitamins although the FDA does not recognize it as such; therefore, there is no recommended daily allowance set for it. There is a vigorous debate on whether IP6 should be categorized as a vitamin. Drug companies have little incentive to research it, since it is a natural compound but a number of researchers on www.pubmed

are studying it. If you recall, B vitamins are water soluble and are continuously used in the body, and they must be constantly replenished. Remember how critical the B vitamins are for liver and gallbladder health including normal bile salts function and detoxification. Perhaps the most known benefit of the B vitamins is ENERGY. Did you ever hear of a B12 shot for energy? Thus, increased energy is another health benefit of IP6.

IP6 exists both in plant and animal cells. Hope Science uses plant sources to get enough to influence our health. The highest levels are found in corn but for supplements IP6 is often extracted from rice bran. Dr. Vanderlinden's IP6 uses rice bran and is free of corn, dairy, lactose, gluten, soy, sugar, and yeast.

Many of you will just say, "Why can't we get enough IP6 from our diet?" This is a good question. Dr. Vanderlinden used to think that dietary sources alone for IP6 were enough but he said that his education and the past ten years of clinical practice changed his mind. Since, I already discussed the S.A.D. and its shortcomings countless times; I need not repeat it again. When we eat a food containing IP6, the IP6 is bound to protein and must separate itself from it during digested in order to be absorbed. The phytase enzyme in our intestines must do this, but the IP6 will be damaged in the process due to the power of phytase. This will render the IP6 less effective. Experimental rats with mammillary-breast cancer were given AllBran. It was not as effective as pure IP6 that was added to their drinking water. Dr. Vanderlinden uses lycopene as an analogy for IP6. Lycopene in tomato juice is more bioavailable than in whole tomatoes due to it being heated or cooked. Lycopene and IP6 are two rare instances where the benefits given by Mother Nature can be helped by man-made technology.

Since the big three in terms of mortality are cancer, heart disease, and diabetes, let me look at the role of IP6 in the latter two. I also mentioned osteoporosis in an earlier chapter as a side effect of the drugs I talked about. I will now discuss how IP6 helps this debilitating problem.

Cardiovascular or heart disease is killing more Americans than any other disease. The research to prevent it has mostly studied cholesterol and blood pressure management. Statins are the main choice for cholesterol in the medical community, but legitimacy is finally to being questioned. Statins lower cholesterol but as I have repeatedly stated, the problem is the inflammation of the arteries, making plaque build-up in the interior artery walls. This build- up is unstable and more prone to break off during normal blood circulation. IP6 has been shown to lower inflammation in other unrelated studies, but since it is a powerful antioxidant, it has the potential to prevent plaque from being built up in the first place. Remember, the inner artery walls need to be injured from the inflammation for them to be repaired with a cholesterol plaque. If the lining of the artery can maintain a healthy status then there will be no plaque build-up and, therefore, fewer heart attacks and stroke. Researchers have found IP6's antioxidant properties protect the heart after the blood supply has been restored. Heart attacks or stroke occurs due to a blockage of blood which then results in a loss of oxygen. Tissues need blood and oxygen at all times, but when the blood supply is restored, let's say after a heart attack, the heart muscle can be damaged from the potent oxidants in the blood. The studies done on animals showed that when given IP6 and induced in them a heart attack, and then allowed, the blood supply to return, these animals had a "very significant protective effect compared to controls." Dr. Vanderlinden thinks that when IP6's binding of heavy metals and calcifications in arteries can be proven in humans, the drug companies will form a super drug. We will no longer pay for a concentrate from rice bran, the current and natural IP6 form; instead the company's drug will be touted as a super drug in the cardiovascular lifesaving category and will be more expensive than statins. I hope for all of our sakes he is wrong because based on the statins's success and side effects, this drug would sell like hotcakes and probably do more harm than good because of its synthetic make-up and probable side effects inherit in drugs.

Let's review some of this extremely important information from the heavy metal section. I said that rock forms of iron from white flour can also interfere with tyrosine absorption affecting the thyroid and adrenal glands. This inorganic iron can also cause LDL and HDL cholesterol to oxidize. LDL and HDL usually form as insulators on the brain and spinal cord, enabling the neural impulses to travel quickly. This is just another example of how cholesterol is so vital for life. When this oxidizes, it causes nerve cells to die, closely paralleling the cell death seen in excitotoxicity. This represents a possible link to neurodegenerative diseases like ALS (Amyotrophic Lateral Sclerosis). When aluminum is bound to the excitotoxins aspartate and/or glutamate (monosodium glutamate), its entry and concentration into your brain is significantly elevated. Once in the brain, aluminum increases iron induced free radical activity. IP6 can also act as a chelator which means to bind. It can chelate or bind iron and aluminum and remove them from our bodies. Can you see how all of this information is interconnected? At bottom, it all comes down to free radicals trying to suck the life out of us.

There are about 17 million diabetic Americans today. 400,000 of these will die each year. Over 90% of these cases suffer from Type II or adult onset sugar diabetes. **This is a travesty since it usually can be controlled with diet and exercise**. New research has found that IP6 is necessary for the process of insulin secretion to occur. It acts like a catalyst in the "stimulus secretion coupling process." What a mouthful that is. It just means that IP6 is one of the crucial substances necessary for the beta cells of the pancreas to secrete insulin. Glucose is what our body uses to make ATP, the energy for our bodies like gas for a car. Remember the K-LASER works by speeding up how fast the body makes ATP. Glucose and inositol, or the "I" in IP6, are linked. Glucose is the mother of inositol which is the mother of IP6. You need to get the glucose from your food into your cells for nourishment and to make ATP. This process requires both insulin and phosphates, of which IP6 provides six.

Osteoporosis is a debilitating disease that affects so many people. A major impact on bone health is digestion. I hear about how much calcium patients take daily so that "there is no way they have osteoporosis." Research shows that even if the person's diet was optimal, only about 1/5 or 20% of the calcium taken would be absorbed. It goes reduces to 5% with the S.A.D. Thus, someone taking 1500mg of calcium may be only absorbing about 60 mg. The answer is chelated minerals. IP6 is chelated. In Cal Mag IP6, the Cal Mag is bound to the IP6 molecule which is considered the "ride in" as Dr. Vanderlinden puts it. (Again Cal Mag ip6 is what I have been talking about this whole chapter. It is just easier to type only the IP6 part.)

IP6 also provides benefits for depression due to its tranquilizing anti-anxiety effect of the inositol. Clinical trials have found it useful for clinical depression, obsessive compulsive disorder, and panic disorder.

There is also a reduction in kidney stone formation with IP6. The mechanism here is the chelation process in which the IP6 binds to the excess calcium and exits the body through the urine. About 1-3% of the IP6 will leave the body through the urine and bind with some calcium from a stone. It chips away at it, so to speak, until the stone eventually dissolves.

IP6 has the perfect ratio of calcium to magnesium atoms or 4:2. Premier Research Labs, which I will discuss next, also offer a high quality mineral supplement from Sango marine coral, which also has a 2:1 calcium magnesium ratio.

Again, you can get Dr. Vanderlinden's book *"Too Good to Be True"* about Inositol + Cal Mag IP6 and decide its value. Many of the best minds in the nutrition world currently endorse and use this product and have deemed it the "Natural Product of the Decade."

The recommended dosage form Hope Science is to take two pills, twice per day for a total of four capsules per day. Each bottle contains 240 capsules or enough for two month's maintenance.

I will discuss the other flagship product known as Essential Fatty Acid Complex or EFAC. Esterification is a chemical processes often involving an alcohol and an acid in the presence of a dehydrating agent for you chemistry buffs. It comes in a cream and in capsules. The theory is that the skin will absorb the cream from the "outside in" allowing the oils to reach the sore muscles and joints while the capsules will work systemically or from the "inside out." Thus you will have "dual absorption" for maximum results.

Glucosamine was the "big dog" in the nineties but looking back at some of the studies; it was really marketing hype that sold it. In an NIH trial, 1,583 patients were studied at 16 different Universities in the most rigorous study of glucosamine ever conducted. Along with Chondroitin or cartilage, these two were taken together since they were supposed to have a synergistic relationship in which they would enhance each other. In this trial there were six groups: two taking glucosamine only, 2 taking a chondroitin only and finally 2 taking a combination of the two. There were also 2 Celebrex groups and two placebo groups.

The results showed that 5 of 6 groups failed to show any benefit over the placebo for pain after a six month period. The group that showed any benefits only contained 72 participants which was less than 5% of the 1583 participants. The researchers also monitored joint and cartilage loss for a two year period. When they measured the joint space, no significant difference was found between the glucosamine/chondroitin groups versus the placebo. In fact there was more of a loss in joint space and cartilage, even though insignificant, however, not beneficial. Thus, the problem is that the advertisers of glucosamine only mentioned these 72 people who reported less pain but failed to mention the other 95% of the participants who had more pain and more loss of cartilage and joint space. This is another good example of deceptive advertising at its finest. For those people who do report good results from chondroitin/glucosamine- that is great. However, EFAC should give you even better results because it is all about ABSORPTION. Glucosamine received a US patent based on research done in 1980- old technology and an obsolete product. It is 2014 and science has come a long way. How does EFAC work? There is a process called an "inflammatory cascade" that Dr. Vanderlinden talks about. The EFAC oils inhibit the chemicals that cause inflammation or receptor inhibition.

In a trial using the EFAC cream published in the Journal of Rheumatology, participants were tested before applying the cream, 30 minutes after the first application, and then 30 days after applying the cream twice daily. The objective criteria here were the following: range of motion (how far could they move), ability to go up or down stairs, ease of getting up from a seated position, and balance when stepping down. The subjective parameter of the study was pain. The results were that after 30 minutes, pain levels were decreased, and the ability to perform the objective criteria tasks improved after a single application. After 30 days, patients improved after applying the cream twice daily and, therefore showed long-term benefits. University of Minnesota researchers found that 95% of esterified oils were found to be absorbed. Concurrently, it was found that a high concentration of the oil was found in the white blood cell membranes. Significantly, white blood cells are found in a high concentration at sites of injury and inflammation. A very important point with EFAC is that researchers found it in all of the same tissues whether applied topically with cream or systemically with capsules. This means true absorption.

In a study done at Scripp's Conference in San Diego in 2007, EFAC was given to 93 osteoarthritic patients. Researchers measured objective data, i.e. how far patients could walk in six minutes. Subjective data consisted of a pain scale. Walking distance improved after just 2 weeks and improved with each testing. The distance walked before EFAC went from an average of 233 feet to 330 feet after 4 weeks and 537 feet after 9 weeks. There was no change in the placebo group.

Dr. Vanderlinden's father broke his heel 18 years ago. He took MSM, glucosamine, and ate a lot of fish oils from the salmon in his diet. He still had to drag his foot due to the heel pain if direct pressure was applied, and he could only walk 2-3 blocks at a time. Incredibly, after taking EFAC for 30 days his father was walking 3-4 miles at a time, something he had not done that in over 10 years. For the first thirty days he only used the cream and then only used the capsules. Incidentally, rubbing the cream in his foot also helped the arthritis in his hands. Dr. Vanderlinden stated, "This was a dramatic improvement in the quality of my father's life."

Here is a finding that is absolutely incredible. In another study, an internist gave 10 family members EFAC capsules, three of whom were scheduled for a knee replacement. All ten improved and had less pain and two out of the three were taken off the surgical list!

Another patient suffering from peripheral neuropathy, developed after a bad lower back injury in 1999, had a burning sensation and pins and needles that could not even be remedied by heavy narcotic pain medication. He would had to go to the hospital for an intravenous drip of morphine 3-5 days a week to get any type of relief. After the first time he applied the EFAC cream to his feet, within 15 minutes he had a massive pain reduction in his feet bringing him to tears of joy that something actually helped his pain.

EFAC is also great for animals. There are many testimonials of dogs that were scheduled to be euthanized due to their inability to walk. Within a week many of them made a miraculous turn around and stayed mobile even at advanced age.

Along with arthritis, fibromyalgia is another condition for which many patients have benefited immensely from EFAC. As Dr. Vanderlinden puts it, "It's all about the inflammation." Almost all disease and pathology is related to inflammation, even the process of aging. Just like the orthopedic and neurosurgeon used to say when dealing with back and neck disk injuries, "Whoever manages motor function, owns the case." Now when it comes to overall health and wellness I would say whoever manages overall body inflammation is going to own the case.

Obviously, safety is of utmost or paramount importance when dealing with any product. University of Minnesota researchers fed rats 1300 times the recommended EFAC dose and still no pathology was found. This would be the equivalent of a person taking almost 4000 capsules per day. Dr. Vanderlinden stated that so far there have been over a billion doses of EFAC taken without incident. So here are the recommendations for EFAC cream and capsules in terms of dosage.

In my practice, I use both the cream for acute and chronic pain and the capsules for inflammation that usually accompanies the pain. (Note: I recently found out that the cream has parabans in it. Obviously Dr. Vanderlinden feels they are safe or he would not have put them in his formula. He even defends parabans as being beneficial in some ways and said that he formed his company partly to find a natural cancer prevention alternative due to his family history. However, since I am trying to offer products to my patients who are "excipient-free" I chose to not use the cream anymore. If a patient requests it, they can get it. A former worker from Hope Science formed a company called Elite Science who offers the same cream with no parabans and the same pills under a different name of 1-TDC which is 1-Tetradecanol complex). You will find out shortly that parabans are a carcinogen; therefore, I will not be buying or using the cream. The capsules are also for lubrication of the joints, and both Hope Science and Elite Science sell the capsules. There are 90-120 capsules per bottle depending on which company they are from. Here is the dose that Hope/Elite science recommends for maximum results. I concur and have been doing it with my patients. First is the loading phase, the first month of treatment during which the patient takes 9 capsules per day. I have most patients take two pills with meals three times per day saturating the body systemically or internally. After the first month the maintenance dose is 3 capsules per day with meals. Each bottle of EFAC or 1-TDC contains 90-120 capsules. Thus, your first bottle lasts 10 to 13 days and with the maintenance dose of three per day, each bottle will last a month to forty days. We are currently telling patients to rub the Elite Science brand cream in twice per day over the involved area(s) or just break open two of either brand capsules per day and rub them into affected area for one month along with swallowing the capsule dose to get the "outside in-inside out" saturation with the body. You will of course use more capsules this way and must take that into account. The capsules are more potent than the cream but many patients do not want to be bothered with cutting off the end and rubbing the gel in. Either way is fine.

CHAPTER FOURTEEN

The Metabolic Way to Health: Premier Research Labs

Again, I cannot thank Dr. Mike Johnson and Dr. Kevin Connors for introducing me to PRL. Their products are incredible and I have had great success with them. There is so much information to cover so I have to scale it down to the bare essentials. First I want to talk about PRL and its founder Dr. Marshall, a PhD biochemist.

Many years ago, Dr. Robert Marshall suffered from tryptophan poisoning almost dying twice. In desperation, he turned to food and whole nutrients to get back to health because traditional medicine had no answers for him. As a result, he ended up creating Premier Research Labs (PRL) and is their current CEO. Dr. Marshall's mission statement is, "To empower every person to access their own limitless healing potential through the use of quantum resonance nutraceutical formulations, spectacular detoxification techniques and premier quality therapeutic strategies..."

Now PRL has been well known internationally for its "excipient-free" nutritional formulations. This means that these products are free of any fillers or binders such as glues or toxic tag-alongs. A handout in my office explains why PRL products are so unique. I don't exactly know which doctor in the Johnson Group developed this handout but whoever the author is, I extend my thanks.

Here are some other fillers, excipients, and toxic tag-alongs present in most supplements brands:

- Magnesium stearate is a cheap lubricating agent. Research shows it can suppress the immune system by suppressing T killer cells

- microcrystalline cellulose is a cheap filler
- Silicon dioxide (common sand) is a cheap flowing agent
- Methyl paraban is a benzoate family member which is known to be a cancer causing agent. (This is what I was referring to above with hope science and the EFAC cream)
- Natural flavors- This is another name for MSG (monosodium glutamate), a well-known neurotoxic agent and excitotoxin
- Methacrylic copolymer/acid- this has been known to be harmful to rat embryos
- Trimethyl citrate- this is a plasticizer
- Titanium oxide- this is used for color and is toxic to the liver
- Corn Starch- typically this is from cheap GMO corn and can elicit allergies
- Talcum powder is a common excipient rarely listed on the label. It is a suspected carcinogen

Tablets always contain excipients due to the way they are made. It requires tons of force to compress them. ***You should NEVER take tablets, ALWAYS take capsules.***

Here are some more questionable agents that are used in both capsules and tablets you may or may not see on the label:
- D&C RED #33
- Propylparaben
- Hydroxyprpyl methylcellulose
- Hydroxyprpyl cellulose
- Polyethylene glycol Red ferric oxide-orange shade
- Methyl p-hydroxybenzoate
- Propyl p hydroxybenzoate
- Sodium acetate
- Sodium metabisulfate
- Eudragit

Why are these excipients added to most nutritional supplements? MONEY is the reason of course. Companies can make the supplements cheaper and quicker with inferior ingredients. Why would you want to take in anything that is not nutritionally beneficial to you and is toxic and damage the cell at the DNA level?

Let's explore some other unique characteristics about PRL nutritionals. Ideal cell resonance is something that may have you baffled. The cell energy principles apply to nutritionals as well as the body. "Quantum coherence" means that the energy field, known as the plasma energy field or the field around the body, must be balanced or coherent.

All of the detriments, I previously discussed in the earlier chapters such as toxins, heavy metals, electromagnetic fields, and many other environmental hazards, affect this balance on the bio- field by depolarizing it. Every cell in our bodies has an outer membrane structure known as a semi-crystalline matrix and each cell resonates at a certain frequency just like a crystal glass that rings a certain note when struck with an object. For the resonant frequency of our body cells to be ideal, we have to consume nutrients that also resonate at the same ideal frequency. Thus when you have a diseased tissues or organ's, it is vital to feed it nutrients whose own frequencies closely match the ideal healthy organs or tissues ideal frequency. This ideal frequency matching is unattainable unless these nutrients have been grown in fertile, rich, unspoiled soil with clean air, water, and natural fertilization-and have been kept free of chemical additives, preservatives, flowing agents, binders, or irradiation. According to Dr. Marshall, to do this we must go to India, South America, and China to tap into their pristine mountaintops for the essential pure ingredients used in the ideal nutritional products. He maintains most US soils are tragically ruined.

Live source products is another unique characteristic of PRL. Nothing that is non-live or inorganic can be good long term for a live or organic source such as the human body. Inorganic or non-live has neither cell resonance nor any DNA. Only some temporary benefit can be found from the biochemical reactions with the inorganic non-live nutrition. Importantly, since there is no DNA in it, there will be no necessary bio-photons (light) to provide to the body cell's DNA.

Vegetable capsules – These capsules are made from tree fiber which is easily digestible safe.

Packed in Violet Containers- This assures maximum protection of the ingredients and high frequency of the cellular resonance.

Produced according to the highest commitment to safety, efficacy and quality- There is no inferior, poorly grown, old toxic raw materials. Each batch arrives and is tested to verify that it meets all strict PRL standards or it is rejected.

It is amusing that on one of my previous orders, I told the PRL consultant that I referred them another chiropractic office that uses a different supplement line. "I told the front desk lady, in the chiropractic office, that if she was going to use supplemental nutrition in their office, you might as well use something that works." The rep started to laugh and said that the PRL motto actually is "Nutrition that really works."

When we are dealing with "quantum coherence" we are dealing with unlimited potential for healing. PRL dispels the old biomechanical model of healing as outdated. That is you take a vitamin to heal the tissue from just the biochemical reaction void of any energy or frequency. I know that this is a bit hard to explain. A book called *"Vibrational Medicine"* written by Richard Gerber MD goes over this in detail when he compares Newtonian physics to Einsteinium physics.

You can go on the website yourself to investigate at www.prlabs.com. Dr. Marshall also has a live radio show as well as an archive of previously recorded shows at www.qnlabs.com.

CHAPTER FIFTEEN

Grocery List of Maintenance Supplements

Here I will discuss what the PRL products are and their use. There is "a grocery list" of nutritional supplements that we should take on a daily basis due to our aging and an adverse environment. In other words, these are my recommended maintenance products. PRL has a whole catalog of other products I also use to treat patients.

To determine the proper balance of the body's pH, the urine must be tested in the morning with a test strip of paper; this is one of the most important things you can do for your health. The first morning urine pH level range should fall between 6.4 and 7.0. This alkaline or basic reading is essential for the body's immune system to function normally. Many researchers will tell you that cancer and most chronic diseases do not survive in an alkaline pH environment.

Most people are acidic due to the S.A.D. This means the reading falls between 5.0 and 6.2. For example, to test pH, a person tests the clean catch first morning (**after 5am**) urine and the test strip indicates a 6.0 reading. The proper procedure is to continue testing it daily for two weeks obtaining an average. The *pH trio* is indicated if the average does not fall between 6.4- 7.0. The problem with acidic pH is that the body will leach calcium from the bones to buffer the blood. We need bone health, not only for skeletal support but to make red blood cells. The S.A.D. is comprised of so much inferior protein that there is little calcium in the diet; moreover our soil is 86% deficient in minerals. Let's return to the example 6.0 pH first morning urine. The body takes the calcium from our bones; this is called microcrystalline hydroxy appetite. Then this calcium has to be re-deposited in the tissues somewhere in the body at the time when it is no longer needed, usually between 5:00 – 7:00 am. Calcium seems to have an affinity for the ears and eyes where it could lead to calcium deposits. Some people with tinnitus or ringing in the ears are experiencing the results of these deposits. Moreover, what this means for many people are that they are losing bone all over. Importantly, the ideal soft tissue reserve, known as mono-ortho-calcium phosphate, will develop by taking the pH trio. Thus, the solution to low or acidic pH is to take the *pH Trio*, consisting of *Aloe Pro, Vitamin D3* drops, and *Coral Legend Plus*. The *Aloe Pro*, should be taken in one to two ounces of water with 6 drops of *Vitamin D3*; each drop of *Vitamin D3* is 1100 international units (iu). The *Coral legend Plus* can be taken in powder or capsule form. I usually give it to patients first in the powder form so they can adjust the dosage with a measuring spoon until the pH reaches 6.4 and stabilizes for a couple of weeks.

Aloe Pro, consisting of the organic inner leaf gel and pulp, is "as close as it gets to eating fresh aloe right in the field," to quote PRL. While most other Aloes are loaded with sodium benzoate damaged from being heated, *Aloe Pro* is made from the Aloe barbadensis species and is an excellent carrier mechanism for the coral legend to reach your soft tissues and form the soft tissue reserve.

Coral Legend Plus, from Sango Marine Coral, is among the cleanest on the planet and is very environmentally protected. Along with Hope Science's IP6, the coral legend has a perfect ratio of 2:1 calcium to magnesium, a key factor in making the pH alkaline or between 6.4 and 7.0 because it is the most bioavailable form. Either *Coral legend Plus* or IP6 is an excellent choice here. Most calcium is junk obtained from a bunch of ground up rocks and is not at all beneficial. Remember, I talked about the necessity of having calcium in the brush border cells of your intestines to deflect and compete with any heavy metals from antiperspirants or processed foods, for example, such as aluminum and mercury. The calcium on the receptor sites prevents these heavy metals from binding. Furthermore, all foods influence pH. Green leafy vegetable and fruits are more basic or alkaline; whereas, meats and highly processed carbs containing a lot of sugar are more acidic, and will lower pH.

Vitamin D3 also enhances the absorption of Calcium and magnesium. Most people are not taking the right kind of Vit D3, however, if taking any at all, recall that I said just about everybody is autoimmune with today's S.A.D.? What calms down an autoimmune reaction is live source Vit D3. Most of the population is deficient in this important vitamin because gallbladder and liver issues restrict its absorption.

Blood sugar health and digestion are other areas that demand balance. I have emphasized that most Americans are not eating right and suffering from reflux and blood sugar imbalance symptoms. First off, most Americans are eating food that is over cooked food reducing the nutritive value. Many nutritionists maintain we should eat more raw foods. Dr. Marshall contends that our bodies are engineered to eat raw food. Thus, by the 30s many of us develop increased amounts of reflux and gas, both markers of the inability to digest food. So how can we get any nutrients from food if we cannot properly digest it? Bugs (bacteria) seem to set up house in the circulatory blood vessels system. If one cannot properly digest food, it rots all of the way from the gastrointestinal tract to the anus disrupting the local bacterial ecology in the gut and challenging the immune system. This will also leave one fatigued or tired. So what is indicated then for someone over 30 years old? I recommend digestive enzymes, in particular, *Premier Digest.*

These pancreatic enzymes should be taken with every meal. Normally the pancreas releases protease to digest proteins, amylase to digest carbohydrates, and lipase to digest fats. When one is over 30, you do not produce enough of these enzymes, consequently, when you eat cooked foods like meat, you cannot fully absorb the protein. These enzymes also make the hydrochloric acid work better. Never eat a meal of cooked food without these enzymes. The dose is based on bodyweight.

Premier HCL - This is hydrochloric acid. Along with *HCL Activator* it is the first line of detoxification in the body. These two components comprise The *"HCl Detox Kit"* from PRL. The body requires HCL to disinfect cooked food. I already explained HCL and its importance in an earlier chapter, but wanted to go into more detail due to its importance in maintaining the very best health possible.

Most people have a lack of stomach acid and, surprisingly not too much, as they often think. Refer to the antacid topic I discussed earlier. The proton pump inhibitors such as Prilosec stop the production of hydrochloric acid in the stomach which damages and stops the digestive process. This low stomach hydrochloric acid state results in undigested food sitting in the stomach and fermenting leading to gas and bloating as the stomach contents putrefy. Lactic acid, a byproduct of incomplete carbohydrate metabolism from bacterial fermentation, is produced from this rotting food which results in the full bloated stomach pushing its contents into the esophagus causing burning. The bloated stomach not only contains the undigested food but also a small amount of hydrochloric acid and copious amounts of lactic acid. Lactic acid can cause burning but it cannot digest food. The stomach is designed for high levels of acid, but the esophagus is not, and the lactic acid causes heart burn. However, by taking proton pump medications, like ant-acids, you are stopping the needed hydrochloric acid production that will prevent the assimilation of proteins, minerals, and vitamins such as B12. The resultant lack of stomach acid also prevents the liver bile from entering the stomach inhibiting digestion of fatty acids. This process also inhibits methylation which will result in deficiencies and chronic health conditions of every kind. **Hypochlorohydria (low stomach acid) is a foundational problem affecting many of our chronic**

patients and is the 1ˢᵗ problem I try to restore. Without the proper stomach acid, the best supplements and diet are useless.

HCL Activator - This is the other half of the HCL detox kit, what re-methylate's the cell or prevents the chronic diseases. It contains potassium and is the carrier mechanism for methylation to the DNA of the cell. The *Premier Digest* is taken first, at the beginning of the meal; the *HCL* and *HCL Activator* are both taken at the end of a meal. Dosage is dependent on bodyweight. The HCL detox kit, is also great for getting rid of the junk, Microcrystalline Hydroxy-appetite, I discussed at length with the pH levels in the previous pages. By using a much higher dose of *HCL* and HCL *Activator*, the body will be able to dissolve and eradicate those unwanted calcium deposits.

As I explained earlier, you CANNOT have good health if either the gallbladder or liver is not functioning properly. I must go into more detail how they are an intricate part of digestion. For those unfortunate people who had their gallbladders removed, supplements will be required.

The gallbladder gets bile from the liver and dumps it in the small intestine. It then precipitates cholesterol from the blood to keep the levels balanced. The bile salts must be prevented from blocking the bile veins or the gallbladder itself. In addition, the liver needs to absorb all of the nutrients it can from food whether only partially digested or rotting in the gut. It then detoxifies any drugs, chemicals or toxins ingested, and dump them into the bile which goes out with the feces.

The MAIN PLAYER in the normal digestive process is vitamin B6, hard to get B6 from supplements since it is not fat soluble. Thus, your body has to make it and stress depletes it. Therefore, PRL has a supplement called *Max Stress B* which provides the N chain form of the B vitamins. Most other B vitamins products are composed of thiamine monohydrate, an inferior form of the vitamin the body does not tolerate and has to "dance" around with. Also this form of B is not methylated. Max Stress B uses only thiamine carboxylate, the fully methylated form that your body wants and also contains the non-flush form of niacin called Niacin Hexanicotinate, which prevents red blood cells from sticking together. It is indicated when clotting occurs and does not respond to blood thinners. It will also strengthen the adrenal glands helping them to hold magnesium in the blood. **It is also an antidote to caffeine.**

If your digestion has been bad for a long time, you are under a lot of stress, or if you are a women who took birth control pill for at least 3 months, chances are that you will have to supplement B6 for the rest of your lives and normal levels may not be enough. Here Dr. Marshall also recommends coffee enemas to get the crud off the liver. This is a procedure that is usually not embraced my most but its health benefits are nothing short of incredible. I will not discuss the coffee enema procedure here, but I do have the recipe for those interested. In his most recent publication, *"You can beat Thyroid Disorders Naturally"*, Dr. Johnson even devotes an entire section to the importance of coffee enemas. *Max Stress B* comes in liquid form; the maintenance dose is half to three quarters of a teaspoon per day.

Along with *Max Stress B* we have *Canadian Golden Honey* and *Camellia Pollen* for liver health. Here you want 2 parts honey to 1 part pollen to enhance the health of the liver and also the reproductive organs with its high concentration in bioflavonoids (water soluble plant pigments). The 2:1 dose equates to 1 teaspoon of honey per day and one half teaspoon of pollen per day. This will also control sweet cravings along with the herb gynmnema sylvestre and a dissolved capsule of Aloe Mannin Fx.

Green Tea ND - This is premier anti-aging, digestive, and immune support supplement. Coming in liquid form, it has one half of a teaspoon serving size containing 103 mg of polyphenols comparable to drinking 20 cups of green tea at one time! The problem with most green teas is their high fluoride content because of the way that their grown, whether organic or not in the US. Green Tea ND is probiotic generated with strong anti-oxidant properties to help regulate the AGE's that I mentioned before when protein molecules bind with sugar molecules. It also offers remarkable support for joint flexibility and also contains 9mg of Resveratrol in a one half teaspoon serving size. This is one of the best products and most valuable for reducing overall body inflammation.

Quinol ND- like Co-enzyme Q-10 (CoQ-10) is the fully reduced form of ubiquinol that helps those body cells too low in energy for regular Co-Q-10 to save them, Co Q-10 on steroids! It can also facilitate the cell's heavy metal and chemical detoxification. It has been clinically tested to provide broad support for the organ/gland systems and brain/attention support. *Quinol ND* was reformulated and it was unavailable until recently.

Premier Greens - I cannot say enough about greens, since mom put an indelible stamp on my head stressing their importance. These vegetables are a live source and contain wheat and barley grass (yes they are gluten free), oat grass, noni, blue green algae, and coriander leaf. Greens are crucial for maintaining an alkaline pH level between 6.4 and 7.0. This is available in powder or capsules and the recommended serving size is two capsules three times per day or one teaspoon mixed in fluids three times per day.

Adaptogen R3 - This formula includes a mushroom blend of the "3 R's": Rhaponticum, Rhodiola Rosea, and Rhodiola Crenulata. It also contains a blend of sea grass and Fo TI blast- a premier botanical revered for centuries. *Adaptogen R3* is known for its hormonal regulation properties by raising or lowering those when needed. Most women- according to their husbands that is, (ha-ha!) could really use this product.

New Zealand Deer Antler - This is premier support for reproductive organs and bladder health for both males and females. It also supports spine, cartilage, and connective tissues such as tendons and ligaments. I remember one patient's husband saying, "Nothing in nature grows as fast as deer antlers." Dose is one pill per day preferably before 2 pm.

EFAC/1-TDC capsules from hope/Elite science and paraban-free 1TDC cream from Elite science - I already described these in detail. To summarize, the capsules are more potent than the cream. If you break open a capsule and apply it to the affected area during the first month saturation phase, you do not even need the cream.

DHA (Docosohexanoic acid) Capsules and EFAs liquid (Essential Fatty acids) - Fatty acid recommendations are currently a volatile topic. It is all over the news that fish oil, which is EPA or Eicopentanoic acid, is not beneficial and could in fact cause prostate cancer. I will extensively discuss the controversy and fatty acids in the last chapter. The main problem with most fish oil has ALWAYS BEEN that it is not good quality and usually turns rancid. For example, according to Dr. Marshall, cod liver oil currently available in the US is not a high grade and may contain mercury or other contaminants which must be removed. Many companies use molecular distillation. In this harmful process, using different molecular weights, they alter the original oils in such a way that the natural beneficial triglycerides are lost. After these altered oils are converted through distillation into ester alcohols, through further distillation they become fatty acids.

Extreme temperatures, as high as 390 degrees Fahrenheit, are used to remove toxins. Solvents such as hexane can be used which can damage fats. In addition, distillation also removes the natural

Vitamin D and Vitamin A. Does it make sense to use a toxin to remove other toxins? It certainly does not sound like to good science to me. In the end you are left with something that CAUSES OXIDATION by damaging the cells instead of healing them totally negating the fish oils main purpose. On the other hand, natural fish oils, which have not been distilled, still may contain mercury or other contaminants and are not recommended.

The plant based algae DHA, for example, is collected right from the source. In other words it did not have to be eaten by a fish along with any toxins. DHA constitutes 15 -20% or so of the human brain, 30-60% of the human retina, and is located in great amounts in various nerve cells throughout the body. If the DHA levels in the body were to approach zero, a person would suffer from neurological problems such as a lack of coordination, and over time more serious neurological deficits including reduced brain volume, learning ability, and memory.

When using QRA muscle testing, Dr. Marshall has found marine source omega 3 oil supplements generally test poorly. This means they have a bad effect on some organ or gland and are not wanted by the body. An exception to this is algae derived DHA.

Dr. Marshall further explains that when we look at the nutritional research over the past twenty years, the single most important factor in improving human health and combating chronic disease is an increased dietary intake of Omega-3 fatty acids in which most Americans are deficient. Thus, due to its outstanding clinical benefits, a plant source DHA is recommended, because our bodies can then convert the DHA to EPA in the liver as needed.

PRL has plant based DHA and Essential fatty acids which are from organically grown Flax oil. The essential fatty acids also contain unrefined olive oil, unrefined sesame seed oil, and unrefined borage oil. They are also cold pressed and nitrogen flushed to prevent increased peroxidation from oxygen. Again, the body will convert flax oil to EPA and DHA. The recommend dose of DHA capsules is 1000 mg per day with the liquid EFAs serving size two teaspoons per day. You will have to investigate some of this on your own as everybody has an opinion. The main concern is the purity of the oil.

There are a few supplements here that are to be taken when beginning to feel sick, is going to have surgery, or is about to run a marathon. They are indicated in situations that tax or compromise the immune system. So they are not truly maintenance supplements, but they are incredible at kicking an infection before it becomes full blown. I have had ill patients for whom previous treatments where ineffective, for example, bronchitis. I gave the following supplements to them and found they indeed "kicked" the infection for good within a week! Here they are:

Nucleoimmune is the first supplement. Six billion cells make up one nucleotide. A nucleotide is a group of molecules that when linked together, form the building blocks of RNA and DNA. In other words these are the raw materials for the cells that make up our bodies. These are usually stored in the liver and bowel. You definitely want reserves of them. The dose will be condition and situation dependent.

Aloe Mannin Fx- this comes from Aloe barbadensis, grown on volcanic soil and rich in the key compound, acemannan. This really promotes immunity by focusing on mucus membranes. It tries to get the toxins out of the neck, head, and face by making the nose run. It really is a roto-rooter of all the mucus membranes in the body especially the gut. Recent In vitro studies showed this supplement inhibited HIV replication.

Well, that is my grocery list of "maintenance" supplements, give or take a few. Of course this is subject to modification, as new, more effective supplements frequently come on the market. Keep in mind that PRL has a catalogue of supplements for all health concerns.

CHAPTER SIXTEEN

QRA
(Quantam Reflex Analysis)

During his thirty years of intensive research, Dr. Marshall also developed the world's first comprehensive practitioner-assessment technology called QRA, "that allows the practitioner to assess the dynamic status of the human bio-field in order to rapidly restore quantum coherence, the true anti-aging technology underlying limitless healing." QRA "is a simple, safe, and effective assessment tool for analyzing the body's bio-field, its reflex patterns and its nutritional needs." QRA uses special kinesiological testing called a modified digital O-ring technique. The patient applies a firm touch to certain acupuncture points with the index and third digit of one hand, while the other hand is tested using the bidigital O-ring. Here the patient attempts to hold the first and fourth finger together against resistance. If the point is weak or off, this bidigital O-ring will be weak when tested. A firm touch is used so we are assessing the patient's meridian system. Remember from the NanoSRT section, that meridians are highly organized networks of interconnected bio-energy pathways which correspond to various organs and glands.

Again, like the NanoSRT I discussed previously, this is an energy technique and is based on 3000 year old acupuncture principles that have proven to be true. I was trained in a level one QRA seminar and use this technique in my office. So what does this mean? Using the QRA technique, I can determine what nutritional products your body needs or does not need. So let's say one of the acupuncture points tests off or weak. QRA then has a list of nutritional products which are ranked from the "best" choice to "other" choices. We then place an apron on the patient and put the indicated nutrition in his apron which is in his bio-field. I then do the bidigital O-ring test to see if he hold strong or weak. In other words, does the nutrition turn off or on the previously tested weak point(s)?

Now along with testing your body on its nutrition needs, QRA also provides a method to assess old traumas to see if they are affecting organs and glands. Think of it this way. There is a light that radiates around our outer shell, resonates, if you will. A surgical scar or trauma will causes a break or interference in this energy field. This interference of energy flow can then affect some organ causing a depolarizing effect. The goal is to repolarize or balance the flow of energy between the brain and all of the organs or glands. Here is an example of how this works: a patient comes with a chief concern or complaint. I will look at any trauma, surgery, scars, or dental fillings, etc., he has had and test him using the bidigital O-ring test to find out if there is an interference field. I check each one of the above suspects until I find an interference field. Once I found that there is an interference field, I check the nearest command center point to see if the interference field is reflexing to one of the organs or glands in the body. There are eight command centers on the front of the body which run along the gallbladder meridian, or the exact center of the body, from the pubic region to the top of the head. There are eight on the back of the body in the same exact spots. I don't want to get too in-depth with this explanation as I know this may sound too esoteric to many skeptics. I have seen too many results using kinesiology to not fully believe in it-when, applied correctly this. There some unscrupulous doctors and unlicensed "practitioners "who will not be objective and simply want to sell vitamins. I would not want to be a patient of one of these unethical "practitioners".

Applying mud is the next step. Yes, you read it correctly; I am talking about mud as a detoxifying agent. I recommend mudding or applying the mud packs to the four downloads also known as the hands and feet first. Because they are major detoxification centers, PRL offers different types of mud to rid the body of any toxins that have accumulated in the scar or trauma. When you have an interruption of energy flow there will be a build -up of toxins in the system, thus the free energy flow must be restored and the body repolarized so that the energy can flow freely all over the body. The most common mudpack used is the *"Medi –Body Pack"* from some of the purest soil on the planet and contains premium grade volcanic and Kaolin Clays, Peat Magma, Shilajit, and cleansing herbs. After mudding the downloads, if we find an interference field we also apply mud to that point and the organ or gland that it reflexed to. We then just mud the actual interference field point next with another pack known as the *"Magma Pack"*. The first mudpack or *Medi-Body Pack* is used to "help reintegrate the interference field area back into the body's normal theorized energy flow." The second or *Magma Pack* is done to "nourish the target interference field area that was just repolarized." The more toxins we remove from the body the better chance we have to achieve a balanced energy field and better health. After the area is mud packed, we re-test to ensure the point now tests "on" or strong.

I will explain some common conditions people present with and what the PRL products recommended are. Some patients will use the nutritional products like a "cook book", much like the way you take a drug for symptoms. Those at PRL quote their motto for this situation, "At least use something that works". If you take supplements without testing to see what you need, that is ok, but if you are not tested you do not know what your body really needs. If one of my patients, upon testing, does not show a weakness in the bio- field, I still recommend many of the "grocery list" products I discussed due to all of the toxins in the environment and diet that are all around us.

Keep in mind, for patients with any nutritional problems or concerns, I start them off with pH monitoring and put them on the *pH trio* if the pH is not between 6.4 and 7.0. This, along with the foundational testing and the appropriate nutrition, may alleviate or get rid of many of the patient's symptoms before we had a chance to even address them.

Here are examples of conditions that are very common now and how I approach them after the foundational testing. An inability to sleep is a common complaint. There is a sleep point in QRA just behind the ear and down on the mastoid bone that I test to see if the patient needs any indicated nutrition. PRL offers *Tranquinol* and *Melatonin ND* for the right and left sleep point if either tests off or weak. The ND product line from PRL also provides has extra immune support. Again, none of its products are made from animal glandulars because animal cells, although once a live source, do not resonate as much as human cells; our bodies do not want to accept them. Synthetic forms of, let's say melatonin contain inorganic or non-living ingredients with no resonance. Therefore, our bodies do not want to take it in. Keep in mind the body is highly receptive to all of PRL's products. This is HUGELY IMPORTANT.

The inability to sleep may also be caused by a malfunctioning gallbladder. If the gallbladder point is weak the necessary nutrition recommended is *Gallbladder ND*. Many patients may fall sleep easily but then wake up at 2:00 or 3:00 in the morning for no apparent reason. This is usually due to the stomach. So, we test the stomach point for the *HCL Detox kit*. If the point is off, I suggest the *HCL Detox kit* along with *Digest*.

Many people also wake up to urinate several times. Here we test the bladder and uterus/prostate points. If these are off we may test for *Ultrapollen*. Some people also feel fatigued or not well rested after they wake up. Here I may test for *Adaptogen*. Thus all of these supplements may be involved in the treatment for sleep problems. Often times I will start with one supplement and add to it if indicated.

I also use stress tapping when I suspect any immune stress. After testing a weak point turned on with the appropriate nutrition in the patient's apron and bio-field, I stress tap it or tap the point four times to see if, the indicated nutritional remedy holds up to my additional stress. If the point goes weak, it indicates something stronger is needed. Then I will test for an immune based formula.

PMS or "premenstrual syndrome" is continually a big problem. Dr. Marshall feels that it is due to the liver's inability to conjugate or breakdown unopposed estrogen. With peri-menopause, women also have a lot of similar PMS symptoms such as hot flashes. Here the problem is too much of a certain type of estrogen. The answer is usually digestion. Let's say we do not test because a patient just wants try some nutrition based on her symptoms. With PMS I would give the patient the *HCL Detox kit, Greens, Coral Legend Plus*, and *DHA* or *Premier Essential fatty acids*. If these do not work, I would then go with *Rejuvenation Cream* which has progesterone to balance the estrogen. Usually with peri-menopause and hot flashes, the liver is also involved; I would then try *Max Stress B*.

Hypothyroidism is probably the most popular undiagnosed condition today affecting over 27-30 million women in this country. I made reference to the reasons earlier. I need to spend some time on this one because so many women tell me, "My family doctor checked my thyroid and it is fine." The truth is that the lab ranges your medical doctors use are too broad. Their "normal range" for TSH or Thyroid Stimulating Hormone is .35-5.0. This number is the pathological range. In other words you have a big problem once the numbers hit that range. THIS IS WHY SO MANY WOMEN FEEL TERRIBLE WHO FALL INTO THIS RANGE. On the other hand, the optimal or functional healthy range should be between 1.8 and 3.0. Once your range is above 5.0 your doctor will put you on synthetic hormone and from that point on your thyroid will fail to make any thyroid hormone on its own, and you will be dependent on the thyroid hormone for the rest of your life.

When you fall into this ".35 - 5.0 normal range", your medical doctor will tell you, "There is nothing wrong with you, and it's all in your head." You are still having the normal thyroid symptoms of hair loss, brain fog, and extreme fatigue. We both know "normal" does not include these symptoms. The problem is however, that your TSH may be 4.0 or 4.2. In other words, you are not between the healthy functional range of 1.8-3.0 but, well within the .35-5.0 pathological range. Usually the medical doctor will only order this test but sometimes he will also order T3 or T4. Optimally, these other thyroid tests need to be run if you want to know exactly how the thyroid is functioning. Dr. Johnson wrote an entire book on the thyroid now available that goes into detail on this important gland. Please refer to *"You Can Beat Thyroid Conditions Naturally"*!

I also want mention here that most people suffering from thyroid problems are auto-immune. In fact it is estimated that this number may be 90% or so. How do you know you are auto-immune? First you could be checked for antibodies which would tell you. You can also discover this if your symptoms wax and wane; they seem to go up and down like a roller coaster. One day you feel good and the next bad. The third way to tell if you may be autoimmune is if you are on a truckload of supplements-which may be making you feel worse, by the way. The fourth hint that you are probably autoimmune is that after you became ill with a virus for example, your life totally fell apart. This patient has been to many different doctors who could not find anything wrong. Many other women also develop an autoimmune condition after pregnancy when the T cells of the immune system wrongly switch dominance.

Lastly, If you have a diagnosed thyroid condition that you are taking meds for but still are not feeling good and have to keep increasing your dose to feel better, chances are that more of the thyroid gland is being destroyed or attacked by your body. I may have also pointed out that when the thyroid gland is irradiated surgically removed, some of it will always remain; there is still some tissue left behind. This tissue will then be susceptible to an attack in an auto-immune reaction. It is important to keep this in mind because when I ask women about their thyroid they reply, "It is not an issue anymore since I had mine removed or burned."

QRA protocol for thyroid health is to evaluate the stomach, liver and thyroid points. We also must look at the parathyroid point because it is most susceptible to heavy metal toxicity. Green tea ND is the best product to remedy that. The problem arises, often times, that the parathyroid will sedate or turn off the thyroid making it sluggish or unworkable. A decrease in progesterone can also be the cause of a thyroid problems and it has to be figured in to the equation. So after testing these points, I then test for the indicated nutrition-*HCL Detox kit, Max Stress B, Xenostat* etc.

The point I want to stress here is the interconnectedness of the body systems. Many of these supplements will turn on numerous organ points and thus restore health to numerous conditions. I have to be like a detective trying to figure out which piece is missing or out of order in this human health puzzle.

When I am finish testing the acupuncture points for weakness with the foundation testing and the specific complaint testing, I look at past traumas and scars to make sure they are not interference fields. Let me give you an example. A lot of women complain of weight gained after pregnancy they cannot lose. Their thyroid is probably involved, resulting in a hormone imbalance. Therefore, we test for the indicated nutritionals. However, the problem could be from an episiotomy scar which is right down the center line on the gallbladder meridian. Sometimes, the scar will reflex and sedate or reduce the function of the kidneys and adrenal glands. So we test to make sure the scar is not an interference field, or that it is not reflexing and sedating an organ. Thus we have the patient mud pack the area, take the indicated nutrition, and re-test after a month or so.

Head trauma along the centerline is particularly insidious because the brain point or GV20 for any acupuncture buffs out there is where all of the meridians cross. So scars resulting from past surgeries could be impeding your energy flow and building toxins. To repeat, this then will unfortunately sedate or turn off any organs or glands along that meridian involved.

So in summary, I explained a few examples of conditions I treat with QRA when I test the organ points when allowed by the patient and use symptom based nutritional recommendations for those who do not want to be tested. There are many more protocols I could discuss but that could be a book in itself.

I have also started doing some nutritional QRA testing on a few chronic back and neck patients with no known etiology, during their initial exams. When a patient presents with neck pain for instance, reliable Chinese medicine indicates that there is an imbalance with the gallbladder and or liver flow of energy. With lower back pain, the imbalance is with the kidneys. Thus I will test these acupuncture points and if weak, I will re-test them with the appropriate nutrition that will make these points test on. If they then test strong, I will recommend that the patient should consider taking that needed supplement for their condition. I have found that often times this is the missing piece which solves their neck or lower back pain- both chronic and acute. Also patients who complain of hearing loss usually have some kidney involvement. If we support the kidneys, many times the hearing will improve.

On my website, www.gildeachiropractic.com, I incorporate the NanoSRT with QRA in a 9 visit protocol that has been working well for patients. My short five minute video called is "Functional Nutrition Protocol". I have other five minute videos titled "Importance of pH," "Why are we so sick?", and "Some Conditions Treated." Check these out under video library.

Additional Note: I must mention something I just read on the Johnson forum last week. Dr. Johnson told of a patient afflicted with Lyme's disease who could barely get through the day. She presented to him with a blood test diagnosis from her medical doctor. Dr. Johnson agreed with and confirmed the diagnosis and developed a treatment protocol using kinesiology and something called **Byron White formulas** (www.byronwhiteformulas.com), which are herbal formulas used to treat chronic diseases. These formulas also test on all four polarities as PRL supplements do. The patient was fully active with no pain after only three weeks of treatment! There have been many patients who have even responded to these formulas alone without the need for prescription antibiotics or antifungals. I was so impressed with this protocol; I am going to try these Byron White formulas with some patients I am currently seeing, who also have Lyme's disease. Remember, I do not treat the disease but the patient with the condition.

CHAPTER SEVENTEEN

Achieve Your Ideal Weight

The title of this book is "Health: A Common Sens*ible* Approach." I am sifting through the constant health recommendations and contradictions to find the truth. Now let me emphasize here that most medical practitioners do not have much nutritional training, but they still seem to carry most of the weight with consumer confidence and trust. In other words, the public will go to them more frequently and follow their advice, even though they usually know far less in this field. Now I am making generalizations here. There are some great holistic Medical doctors out there who are well versed in nutrition, but for the most part this is not the case.

When I previously featured the Cardiac surgeon, Dr. Dwight Lundell, I introduced you to this "maverick" eating which means fat is good and sugar and simple carbohydrates are not. I have given most of the information on what types of food to avoid in the beginning section of "why we are so unhealthy." In this chapter I will tell you what foods and their combinations you should eat in order to enhance your metabolic type so that the body can burn unwanted fat.

Each person should find out their metabolic type so that he can eat accordingly. I strongly recommend *"The Metabolic Typing Diet,"* by William Wolcott and Trish Fahey which explains the three types of metabolism: the protein type, the carb type, and the mixed type, which is a combination of the first two. If for example, you have gained too much weight according to the authors, this is a sign of the body's lack of ability to absorb the proper nutrients leading to a constant unsuccessful attempt "to satisfy hunger and normalize metabolism." Remember, that we are biochemically different; different metabolic types demand different food choices.

First we will look at the protein type which means consuming high proteins including the heavy, fatty high proteins, high fats and oils, and lower carbohydrates; sugary foods are not good for this protein type. Next we have the carbohydrate metabolism type, requiring high carbohydrates, low protein, low fats and oils. In other words these two types are exact opposites. There are also pH factors along with cellular oxidation rates and sympathetic/parasympathetic nervous system differences in these types and it gets more complicated than I need to discuss here. To fully investigate metabolic typing, I again refer you to the book. The third type of metabolism is the mixed type in which the body enjoys a combination of the previous two types; there is no sensitivity to carbohydrates or to proteins. Therefore, if you a mixed type you are balanced. Arguably, the mixed types have an easier time keeping their weight stable; they do not have to be as strict with the proteins and carbs by not eating the wrong things as often and altering the metabolic balance. Then of course the stable weight parlays into more stable health and less symptoms.

So here is a statement that I have been harping on for years. **SUGAR IS THE ENEMY- NOT FAT:** Your body will never burn fat if it can burn sugar more easily. Most of you will read this and say that you know candy and sweets are bad, and you avoid them but still feel awful and cannot lose weight. I am not only talking eating pure sugar foods; I am talking about eating the higher glycemic index foods from which the food turns to sugar immediately. Remember, the form of sugar, glucose is what your body turns all foods into so we can burn it for energy. We absolutely must choose foods that slowly turn into glucose so that you have more energy. When you light a fire, you want the kindling to ignite it, but you want the longest slow burning logs to maintain it, right? This is how you should also view carbohydrates. When you are a mixed metabolism type you can get away with more of the higher glycemic foods since you are not as sensitive to them as the other metabolic types, but they still are not as healthy due to the high sugar content and should be eaten in moderation.

Let's look at some foods, such as wheat bread, disguised as health foods. Like many of you, until I learned about the evils of gluten and the havoc it wreaks on our system, I always recommended whole wheat flours. Besides the wheat, there are "low fat" or "fruit juice sweetened" muffins, pastries, cakes, and cold cereals that claim all sorts of health benefits. One cereal commercial claims it will help to "lower your cholesterol." Cold cereals are junk, highly processed and loaded with hidden sugars and chemicals as most salad dressings and condiments are. For example, one cup of honey nut cheerios has as much sugar in it as three Chips Ahoy cookies! The problem with all of these so called health foods is that they will ALTER YOUR BLOOD SUGAR LEVELS IMMEDIATELY. A short while ago my father told me about a study involving the blood sugar levels of people eating bread versus a snickers bar. After an hour they took a blood sample of five of them. Three of those who just ate the toast had the highest levels of sugar in their blood. It was HIGHER THAN THE SNICKERS BAR. So keep this in mind folks, your body does not know the difference between a piece of bread and a candy bar when it comes to sugar content. I hope this also does not make people who usually eat bread eat snickers bars instead?

Ezekiel, sprouted bread, made from rice flour or spelt will not put you in the fat storage blood sugar range. Make sure your bread is also gluten free. Rice is a great grain that will not spike your blood sugar but make sure it is brown rice and not pre-cooked; it should take 40 minutes or so to cook. There was some recent talk about rice having dangerous levels of arsenic in it due to our soil. There was some recent concern that rice contains dangerous levels of arsenic because of our soil. The truth is arsenic is organically bound but not biologically available so although it is bound to the cells, it is inert and inactive thus not causing any problems. Some people, however, are sensitive to it and can have a blood test to determine this from Cyrex labs. Quinoa, pronounced Keen- wah, another grain made from corn is very versatile, like rice, and can be used in many dishes. Remember to get non GMO corn. Although natural and beneficial, fruits must be carefully chosen and eaten in moderation because many of them have high sugar content. Keep in mind you can drink too much freshly squeezed fruit juice thinking you are not spiking your blood sugar. It may take 5 oranges or apples to make 8 ounces of orange or apple juice, but a person would never eat 5 oranges or apples at one sitting. Stone fruits, or pitted ones, have the lowest sugar content. Be careful with very ripe bananas because they eventually will turn to sugar if you let them ripen too long. Apples are the best for maintaining stable blood sugar. The malic acid in apples is also good for other things as well such as chronic fatigue syndrome, fibromyalgia, metal toxicity, oral hygiene, and skin conditions. I guess the apple a day keeping the doctor away is true after all. A great snack is organic almond butter on apple slices. You get protein, fat, and fiber with minimal sugars.

Vegetables are a great source of the necessary valuable complex carbohydrates. I am not talking about peas and corn here; their nutritional value is not great compared to green leafy vegetables or cruciferous ones, like broccoli one of the best cruciferous (leaves resemble a cross) vegetables for health and healthy blood sugar. There is also something in fruits and veggies called fiber that I will discuss soon.

The blood sugar levels in your body are very precise. In other words, there is not a lot of wiggle room in terms of just right, too much or too little. When it is balanced you will feel great, when low you will feel tired with constant hunger and sugar cravings leading to weight gain. The functional ranges of a healthy blood sugar are 85-99mg/dl, also the fat burning zone. Medical doctors shoot for 120mg/dl or less but this is too high and is the weight gain zone. Previously, I discussed how too much insulin being secreted results in more stored fat. Remember, the insulin merry go round where the excessive long-term high blood sugar triggers the release of excessive insulin which actually turns the blood sugar from high to low. The result is exhaustion and inability to achieve the ideal weight. The key here is to release just the right amount of insulin so your blood sugar is balanced throughout the day. In order to do this, we have to know what foods to eat and, MORE IMPORTANTLY, what foods to avoid. Since all carbohydrates are not created equal, the good complex carbohydrates, which have a low glycemic index and do not turn to sugar quickly. But the breads, pastas, and anything and everything breaded, will push your blood sugar in the 120mg/dl and over category which is the fat storage and fatigued mode.

Let me review the glycemic index for those of you who do not remember or understand it. This index is a numerical scale that ranks foods and beverages on their potential to raise your blood sugar and insulin levels. Foods and beverages that rank above 70 are considered high "GI." These are more likely to raise your blood sugar rapidly. Those that fall below 55 are considered low "GI" foods and are not likely to raise your blood sugar levels by any significant amount. There also is the glycemic load. This represents the amount of fiber in a food. Fiber will slow a food down to make up for a higher glycemic index. For example, carrots have a glycemic index of 47 plus or minus 16. But their glycemic load is only 3. The way to determine the glycemic load is: (GI) x (grams of carbs-grams of fiber) divided by 100. Bananas are another food with a glycemic index of 52, but when you figure the fiber into the equation it brings down the glycemic load to 24. This is true with almost any fruits if you eat them whole. When you drink fruit juice, even if pure, you are not getting the fiber and the sugar content is very high. Of course this is not the case if you are using the new bullet juicer, vitamix or Ninja, in which you throw in the whole fruit. Natural food is always better than processed. Your body will be healthier and burn fat for fuel when you eat more fruits and vegetables and much less processed food.

DO NOT DRINK TAP WATER. Remember when I went over fluoride in an earlier section? Fluoride and its partner in crime, chlorine competes with the iodine molecule in the thyroid gland. The rocket fuel ingredient endocrine disrupter, perchlorate, I talked about earlier also competes with and depletes your body's iodine supply. As I stated repeatedly, there are many people who simply have no energy. The white flour and tap water both contribute to this by sabotaging the thyroid. You need to drink one half of your bodyweight in ounces per day but many people in this country do not drink any water because they do not like the taste. Thus this country has a population that is partially DEHYDRATED. Guess what this means to our adrenal glands? They are stressed and not working correctly. All of those sugary, caffeinated sports drinks and coffees actually dehydrate your body further. Spring water which contains minerals is a better choice. Also be aware of the chemical BPA (Bisphenol A), which can leach out of plastic water bottles; glass bottles prevent this. Be kind to your kidneys; they must filter 2000 liters of blood per day, and they need water! Dr. Johnson recommends a great book all about the necessity of water called *"Water & Salt- the Essence of Life."*

Lastly, we need to discuss fat. From all that I have said thus far, you probably already know that fat has taken a bum rap over the years, starting with all of the cholesterol misinformation. The truth is that **FAT IS NOT THE PROBLEM. FAT WILL NOT MAKE YOU FAT; SUGAR WILL MAKE YOU FAT. HOWEVER, FAT COMBINED WITH SUGAR IS EXTREMELY BAD**. Hopefully, you remember the bad fats you should avoid. First are the trans-fats, for example, in margarines and the complete list of butter substitutes, chemically altered fats that do not go rancid. Even bugs will shun them. Our bodies cannot break them down. Other fats are junk oils such as vegetable and canola, safflower and sunflower, unsaturated and unstable, go rancid as soon as they enter the body. Promoting these dangerous polyunsaturated oils, Big Pharma has done a huge disservice to the public health since the start of the cholesterol, stroke, and heart attack scare media blitz. Statistics prove it. In Dr. Lundell's article, he concluded that the low fat diets killed more than they helped and they ruined and continue to ruin the country's health.

The body needs natural unprocessed fats for fuel. The liver cannot deal with inordinate amounts of white sugar and hydrogenated, chemically altered fat. It cannot filter these chemicals and toxins and break down fats efficiently.

Eating a diet full of all of these processed chemicals will prevent you from achieving your ideal weight. An example of these chemicals is MSG, or NutraSweet, two excitotoxins previously mentioned. STEVIA is the only sweetener you should consume because it does not interfere with your blood sugar levels. Some people dislike its taste, but it is just a matter of getting used to it. Also PRL's *Canadian golden honey* is pure and can be taken for reproductive and liver health; therefore, you could kill two birds with one stone, so to speak. Natural Maple syrup is also good if you get the grade B type which has a lower glycemic index than grade A. Agave nectar and sucralose will adversely affect blood sugar levels and will make you store fat. Additionally, most processed foods marketed as health foods have hidden toxins in them for example; most yogurts contain high fructose corn syrup. All packaged foods and microwaveable meals contain too much sugar and chemicals. Most diet snack bars are also loaded with soy and chemicals. **Try to keep the ingredients down to a minimum and eat whole foods like eggs, fresh vegetables, fruits, wild fish, organic chicken, grass fed beef, avocados, coconut milk,**

coconut oil, olive oil, butter, brown rice, sweet potatoes. I know most people are brainwashed into thinking that coconuts have saturated fat and must be avoided. Nothing can be further from the truth. Let me explain....

A saturated fat is one that has a small degree or amount of unsaturation or double bonds. This means it is saturated with hydrogen molecules. Saturated equals stability; coconut oil and butter are good examples. At any temperature below 76 degrees they are solids but, above that temperature, they are liquids. Monsaturated fats like olive oil contain only one double bond. Polyunsaturated fats like corn and flaxseed oils contain many double bonds. Alpha linoleic acid (omega 6) has two double bonds and alpha linolenic acid (omega 3) is polyunsaturated with three double bonds. *These omega three fatty acids are essential; this mean your body needs them but CANNOT MAKE THEM ON ITS OWN.*

Weeding through the contradictory information on which omega-3s to take is when the fun begins. I must explain some the differences between plants based omega-3s and marine based omega-3s. The omega 3 fatty acids in Fish or krill oil differ from the fatty acids in plant based source of algae; it is longer and bent in terms of molecular shape. Fish contains a combination of DHA and EPA (Eicopentanoic acid) by eating the algae or plant based source. Organisms and mammals adapted to the cold have an abundance of these fatty acids. They prevent the cell membranes from becoming too rigid in the cold, enabling them to absorb oxygen and other nutrients as well as to expel toxins that accumulate.

As I have previously said, DHA comprises 15-20% of the total 60% fat in the brain and 60% of the human retina. Located in nerve cells throughout the body in higher amounts it is essential for quick reaction times, eye-hand coordination, and cognition. A deficiency leads to increased neurological deficits. In an article titled "How to Stop or Slow Down Stroke Damage" Dr. Ronald Grisanti from Functional Medicine University described a recent experiment in which strokes were induced in experimental animals. After they administered DHA to the animals within five hours after the stroke, it "cut the size of the infarct (damaged brain area) by up to 77%."

Our bodies can make DHA from the plant-based omega3, when needed. There has been recent controversy among many in the scientific community who contend that most people cannot efficiently convert DHA to EPA and they would recommend that people just take fish oil. This may be true, according to Dr. Grisanti, for those on statins, calcium channel blockers (high blood pressure medicine), and chemotherapy or are exposed to a lot of phthalates. All of these substances can damage the DHA conversion. There is a fatty acid profile test that can evaluate fatty acid levels. Another dilemma also arises for both vegetarians and availability.

Krill, a relative of shrimp, was the answer for a lot of people; Dr. Mercola is one of them who presently endorses krill oil and swears by marine (ocean) sources of krill oil as superior to fish oil due to its astaxanthin content, a potent antioxidant that is "almost 50 times more than is present in fish oil." He adds that this high astaxanthin content in krill oil prevents it from oxidizing the way fish oil does. Moreover, he states that omega-3s can be found in flaxseed, hemp and chia seeds and a few other foods, but only "the most beneficial form of omega-3-containing two fatty acids, DHA and EPA, essential to fighting and preventing both physical and mental diseases, however, can only be found in fish and krill."

Several years ago, Whole Foods, a natural grocery store chain, was ordered to pull its DHA derived from Krill due to sustainability concerns. Krill was found to be the largest biomass on the planet and was supposed to solve the overfishing threat resulting from the DHA demand but ironically, the decline of animal populations that rely on the krill raised concerns enough for the Commission for the Conservation of Antarctic Living Marine Resources to issue fishing restrictions and quotas.

There is also a controversial link recently found between fish oil and prostate cancer. From the recent perfusion of news coverage on television, you may have heard about it. In a recent study there was a "link" found between men who had a higher concentration of marine based omega-3s in their blood also had a high risk of getting prostate cancer? The majority of the participants in this study, however, did not even use fish oil supplements. Reporters and the media were conveniently equating higher blood levels of DHA with fish oil supplement taking. The DHA levels used in the study were based on a percentage of fatty acids not on an absolute value. This can be very misleading. Let me explain with the following analogy: Would you rather have 50% of Tim's money or 5% of Jill's money? Until you know how much Tim or Jill's money is, those percentages are meaningless. The American Journal of Clinical Nutrition explained in a 2009 commentary that the only time percentage of fatty acid content is "meaningful" is when the total fatty acid content is known for all individuals. This was not the case here. Furthermore, 53% of the subjects in the study who had prostate cancer were smokers. Sixty four percent of the cancer subjects consumed alcohol and 80% of them were obese. This study did not prove causation; it only showed a correlation. Dr. Kristy, a researcher for the study, made a statement that makes him sound like a puppet for Senator Durbin's supplement bill. This bill threatens the supplement industry by giving the FDA more power to regulate supplements as if they were drugs. This would quickly put supplement companies out of business. There are hundreds, if not thousands of studies, which show a how great omega-3s are at preventing chronic diseases and helping one achieve optimum health. One study in the British Journal of Cancer in 2006, showed how the spread of prostate cancer was blocked by omega-3s. I agree with Dr. Marshall from PRL and think marine quality oils are inferior to plant based ones, because it is best to get the omega-3s right from the source.

Now let's go back to the sustainability question of krill. The scientific community decided to go to the source which is algae derived DHA, the microscopic algae which makes the DHA itself. They did not want flax source.

Farmed algae which yields DHA is sustainable and is vegan as well as being eligible for kosher and organic certification. It is pure, however, and free of toxins. Between 1996 and 2001, research was conducted by The Journal of Nutrition. The results were published from research done at various institutions like Brigham and Women's Hospital, the Harvard Medical School, and the Wellness Institute of the Cleveland Clinic showing the health benefits of algae DHA supplementation for combating cardiovascular disease and risk factors such as triglycerides, LDL, and HDL cholesterol. Their conclusion was that DHA from algae is sustainable and can satisfy the demands of consumers, including vegetarians, by fulfilling the well documented health benefits established with omega-3s.

The controversy on coconut oil and what type of fat is the most beneficial continues to rage on in this country. I want to present some very important information from an excellent article written by Lita Lee on coconut oil. She discusses the extensive research on saturated versus unsaturated fats conducted by Dr. G Renig and Dr. Ray, both PhDs that found that butter, olive oil, and coconut oil are the best choices.

They explain that for years these saturated fats were associated with high cholesterol, heart attacks and strokes. The drug companies promoted ads such as "I can't believe it's not butter" to convince the unsuspecting public to buy imitation butter as well as many other polyunsaturated products. The authors could not believe, nor could I after thinking about it, where they found any American eating a high saturated fat diet after so much promotion of low fat diets. I emphatically agree with Dr. Dwight Lundell's position on heart disease and the highly processed commercial non-nutritive foods people have been consuming over the past forty years. According to the recent news, the FDA is banning the use of any trans-fats in foods. They said it would save 20,000 heart attacks. Better late than never I always say. This is a step in the right direction albeit a tiny one.

The researchers had to find populations who ate a high saturated fat diet and were healthy. They found that this is the case in tropical climates such as those from Melanesia and the Yucatan. They found that the subject's thyroids were slightly, not pathologically hyperthyroid or overactive due to the thyroid stimulating effects of a diet high in coconut oil, along with fish and fruit. *Remember the 27-30 million undiagnosed hypothyroid cases now eating a diet of unsaturated fats exclusively and thinking they are doing themselves a favor?*

How do you get away with a diet loaded with unsaturated fat you ask? An example is the Eskimos. Their diet is exclusively cold-water fish, which is omega three linolenic acid containing three double bonds. But these people eat the whole fish, head, brains and all. They get the hormonal benefit and again they exhibit a 25% higher functioning thyroid than Americans. So again they are considered hyperthyroid when using the normal medical parameters. Now this hyper acting thyroid is "pathological" by medical standards yet it allowed the Eskimos to burn unsaturated fats. Thus, the two researchers surmised that if you eat nothing except unsaturated fat but are not an Eskimo you might be in trouble. At least you should be very active if nothing else.

Why is coconut oil so great? As I said, first you have stability. Unsaturated fats when cooked become unstable and go rancid in hours. There is a distinct "stale" taste leftovers have due to this. Dr. Peat feels that fresh saturated fats are no better, however, as they will oxidize quickly once inside the body due to being heated and mixed with oxygen. He found that this is not so with coconut oil even after one year at room temperature. The coconut oil showed no evidence of rancidity even though it has 9% linoleic (omega 6) polyunsaturated fat. He then theorized that coconut oil must have antioxidant properties since it does not go rancid and decreases our need for vitamin E, whereas unsaturated fats depletes our body's vitamin E.

Another benefit of coconut oil is regulating cholesterol through stimulating the thyroid gland. A study in 1981 involving islanders with a diet high in coconut oil showed no adverse effects. Then these same islanders migrated to New Zealand, and they decreased their coconut oil consumption. Their cholesterol, mainly the LDL, increased. Thus, according to Dr. Peat "In the presence of adequate thyroid hormone, the LDL cholesterol is converted by enzymes to the anti-aging steroids pregnenalone, progesterone, and DHEA." The cholesterol is the raw material for these hormones to be manufactured by the body. These hormones are required to help prevent many diseases such as cancer and heart disease and also are needed to prevent obesity and chronic degenerative diseases.

With the thyroid stimulating effects of coconut oil you also get weight loss. In the 1940s farmers tried to use coconut oil to fatten up their cattle. To their chagrin, however, the animals became lean and more active with increased appetite. The farmers then tried hypothyroid drug, which did fatten the animals up, but was found to be a carcinogen. A few years later they discovered that feeding livestock corn and soybeans results in it hypothyroidism.

In 1987, a 50 year old study done by Lim-Sylianco echoed the farmer's results findings coconut oil's anti-cancer effects. "In chemically induced cancers of the colon and breast, coconut oil was by far more protective than unsaturated oils. Thirty two percent of corn oil eaters developed colon cancer versus only three percent who used coconut oil. It has significantly been noted that Albert Schweitzer operated a clinic in South Africa for many years before he saw a single case of cancer. He thought that the European diet adopted by many Africans was the beginning of their increase in cancer.

Lastly, there are the antimicrobial or antibacterial, antiviral, and antiprotozoal effects of one of the components in coconut oil, lauric acid; coconut oil contains 40% of it. This Lauric acid is a potent fighter and even present in breast milk. It also has adverse effects on yeast, bacteria, and fungi disrupting the lipid membranes of pathogenic organisms, inactivating them. There you have some great news on coconut oil.

Cows, given the choice will always prefer grass pastures rather than genetically modified grains. Like us, when they eat foods not designed for them, their body composition changes. This altered composition of unsaturated fat is not good for us and them to ingest and is largely contributing to the unbalanced omega three to six ratio most Americans have, not the ideal 3:1. The average American diet, including this unsaturated cow meat, is something like 20:1. Moreover, grass fed beef is also higher in vitamins, 400% higher in A and E and will not cause Mad Cow Disease.

Let me consider the topic of calories because I always get asked a lot of questions about them. In theory if you dump the garbage/processed foods and eat the healthy foods, you would not have to worry about calories; your metabolism would be balanced. Your appetite would be satisfied; you would not constantly be hungry or have cravings. You would only eat what you need to maintain a healthy weight. In the real world unfortunately people follow the path of least resistance and want magic. Most chronically overweight people want to eat and drink whatever they desire and be able to simply take a pill to lose the excess weight, and maintain the loss. In In general, most of the junk foods people eat today are addictive, a result of their being processing with such ingredients as MSG and hybridized gluten. Therefore, one's appetite is never entirely satisfied; the eating becomes constant. This leads me to my next eye opening statement.

I do not want to be a spoiler but the truth is that **you have to burn more calories than you take in in order to lose weight.** However, when you do, and if you have more muscle on your frame making you an efficient fat burning machine, you can eat more calories and not gain unwanted fat.

Having said that I must stress the importance for everyone to just eat the right foods and forego the wrong ones. Probably nobody would have to resort to the calorie calculator for the long haul. Yes, you may have to be on a limited calorie diet for the short-term to lose the weight, but we are worried about the long-term here or a **lifestyle change.**

My mother was just on the phone with me last night summarizing a woman's diet plan which claims to result in a weight loss of twenty pounds or so over the next one to three months. A spokeswoman on one of the day time talk shows said things like, "Only eat one slice of bread with your sandwich," and, "Load up the lettuce with a little bit of meat," and, "Do not add any creamer to your coffee." She concluded that "This will save you x amount of calories if you do this," etc.... If you added up all of her suggestions, you would be saving 3500 multiplied by 20 or 70,000 calories. On the surface this sound logical and right since a pound of fat contains 3500 calories, but research shows that there are other crucial factors involved in weight loss and calorics. For instance, most people believe that in order to lose a pound of fat you need to burn 3500 calories. This is true in theory; however, age, weight, calorie consumption plus metabolic type are all variables, which will alter the 3500-calorie rule to some degree.

Research from the National institutes of Health confirms that a person losing weight has a slower metabolic rate to account for the weight loss. Remember your body's homeostatic mechanism. It must account for too many calories taken in, as in feast, or too few calories taken in, as in famine. Let's look at how our ancestors lived many years ago. Their body's stored calories whenever they could because famine could subject them to a starvation period at any time. Presently, if someone is losing weight his body is trying to balance itself and account for the reduction in calories. If we pick a 40-year-old man who is reducing his caloric intake by 500 per day, we can expect a loss one pound a week or 24 pounds in six months right? However, due to his age, the computer model predicts that this formula is 25% too generous for the amount of weight lost in 6 months and it predicts closer to 19-20 pounds lost or a 25% reduction in the original prediction.

Here is a good time to mention the diet pre-packaged food plans you see on television. They all have one thing in common, caloric restriction, averaging about 1600 calories per day. Their ingredients consist mainly of processed garbage loaded with sugar, chemicals, and polyunsaturated fats. Because the caloric content is so much lower than what the person's body is used to, he loses weight but most likely regains it. Let's look at caloric trends today versus the 1970s. Between 2000-2008 The JAMA (Journal of the American Medical Association) stated that 68% Americans were considered overweight. In fact they said that 35% of women were obese and 32% of men were obese. They also said Americans in general now have a higher body fat than thirty-seven years ago.

According to the USDA, the average American daily caloric intake has risen from 2,234 in 1970 to 2,757 in 2003. This is 523 more calories per day which "leads to a significant weight gain if these excessive calories are not burned off through physical activity."

"The USDA provides a detailed analysis of average American daily caloric increases. Of the 523 daily calorie increase from 1970 to 2003, 292 calories were from added fats, oils, sugars and sweeteners. Grains accounted for an increase in 188 calories each day. Remember the book "Wheat Belly" I referenced earlier, in which the opiate response in the brain from consuming today's wheat can lead to an additional 440 calories per day in the diet. Compared to 1970, in 2003 Americans also consumed fewer calories from dairy products."

The National Heart Lung and Blood Institute recommend, "Moderately active females consume between 1,800 and 2,200 per day while moderately active adult men require between 2,200 and 2,800 calories each day. If you're overweight, reduce your caloric intake by 500 each day to lose about 1 lb. per week to return to a healthy normal weight."

Since obesity is such a major problem in this country, I want to consider more weight loss strategies including some myths people have about "dieting" that science has disproven. **When it comes to calories there really is no magic.**

Currently many people are confused about whether to eat three versus six meals per day. Most personal trainers tell their clients that they are actually not eating enough or often enough. Since cooking at home demands more time, they often settle for frozen dinners or restaurant take out. Others eat only a few meals per day, but most of which is junk food. Still others may "pig out" at lunch and then eat nothing else after at 8pm. Many nutritionists and athletic trainers recommend the six meals per day diet that maintains proper blood sugar levels without spikes and valleys causing insulin surges leading to fat storage. If you must snack between meals then be careful to JUST snack and keep the portion size to a minimum. Any snacks such as a handful of nuts, an apple or celery sticks with almond butter, and an organic high protein bar, are good choices that would supply only 200-300 calories at most. Be careful to just snack; attempting to lose weight by eating a 500 calorie snack, in addition to regular meals, is a disaster.

Another variation is eating six or seven meals of the same food, which consist of an equal amount of calories. If you are super regimented or are self-employed you would choose a food and determine what a 1200-1600 calorie portion size is and just divide this into six or seven portions, eaten throughout the day. By following this routine, you can eat any time and even on the run. It is likely that this is not something most people would continually follow over a long period because of a lack of variety.

Research has shown that people who only eat three main meals per day are actually no hungrier than those who have more frequent smaller meals. One study done at the University of Missouri found that to reduce the worry about portion control, a better strategy is to just eat three square meals per day. Again, portion size is a huge problem. In too many restaurants you will be given at least two servings on a huge plate; half of which should be eaten and the other half taken home.

Moreover, people who want to eat only one or two meals per day will probably experience too many spikes in their blood sugar levels sabotaging their weight loss goals. Common sense holds that you need a certain amount of food per day that it should be spread out strategically to fit into your work, play, and leisure time in a convenient fashion. This plan should ensure that you will continue eating that way for the long haul; **healthy eating is a LIFESTYLE CHANGE and not a temporary diet plan**.

I must address a few myths that people have believed for years. The first one is that yo-yo dieting hurts your chances for future weight loss. Though it has been proven in rat studies that forced yo-yo dieting made them become more efficient at gaining weight, this is not the case for humans. A study by the Fred Hutchinson Cancer Research Center in Seattle found that a history of losing - gaining, - losing "wasn't linked to any negative side effects on metabolism." This does; however, seem to have an adverse effect on the dieter's mind. After a while, they become disillusioned and just give up entirely. Let me be clear: yo-yo dieting is not good for you, but it also will not prevent you from being able to lose weight in the future.

Another myth concerns exercise and weight loss. Many people believe that you can "eat what you want," and as long as you are active you will not gain weight, and in fact lose weight. This may hold true for those who do not need to lose weight since their muscle to fat ratio is higher, and their fat burning metabolism is in peak shape. But for the majority of those who constantly endure the battle of the bulge, this is not the case. Recent research supports the fact that exercise does not burn off pounds. This is hard to believe and does not sit well with many. The study consisted of 411 women who exercised from one to three hours per week for six months and "didn't lose significantly more weight than those who devoted themselves to sedentary pursuits." Although it sounds flawed, there were 15 other studies conducted that reached the same conclusion: moderate workouts do not lead to weight loss. The researchers theorized that maybe these people who are working out are getting hungrier and eating more. The reason for this conclusion could be the biological answer; the body's homeostatic balance is being compromised. The way our body wants to compensate for more or less calories taken in and burned is by altering the metabolism or the way our bodies process food for fuel. When you exercise, your body compensates by lowering your resting metabolic rate by about 7% so that you burn less calories. The study found this amount to be 50 to 75 fewer calories burned per day. Do not get confused with the resting metabolic rate of someone very muscular. When someone has a lot of muscle on his frame and little fat, his resting metabolic rate will be higher just to feed the large amount of muscle. Workouts aimed at putting on lean muscle will eventually boost your metabolism as you will start to get more muscle. Thus resistance training is key to weight loss by putting more muscle on the body's frame. It is the result of gaining muscle and not the calories burned by lifting the weight itself that leads to weight loss.

Another myth involves drinking milk which some people actually think causes them to lose more weight. **Nothing can be farther from the truth**. You know how I feel about humans drinking cow's milk. A Harvard study revealed that those milk drinkers gained weight. ENUF SAID!

Many other people also think if they just count their carbs, they can keep those unwanted pounds off. Research has found that this is not the case. After studying adults who had recently lost a significant amount of weight, they found that those who restricted carbs caused an increase in cortisol, the adrenal stress hormone, and C-reactive protein, which are measures inflammation in the body. The elevation of these two markers could adversely affect your health, contributing to cardiovascular disease; also, with high cortisol blood sugar regulation problems. Moreover, they found that those who counted fat grams were the least successful; their metabolism slowed down to the point of 423 fewer calories being burned per day. What nutritional plan was the winner? **The balanced plan of course**. There was a less extreme drop in calories burned per day only 300 or so, and there was no elevation of cortisol or C-reactive protein so the heart was happy.

Admittedly there are some rare instances where a person can go on a very restricted caloric diet, even gastric bypass, and still not lose any weight. These patients have metabolic and endocrinological problems which, according to recent research don by Ken Holtorf, MD, involve two particular hormones. In an article posted on the Johnson group board by Dr. Ron Brandied, Dr Holtorf is interviewed and revealed the complexities of weight loss for some unfortunate people. Dr. Holtorf states that leptin and rT3, a Thyroid hormone, are the culprits that need to be evaluated and treated so these patients can lose weight. Leptin is a hormone secreted by fat cells. Dr. Holtorf found a that those weight loss resistant patients who had a high leptin reading also had a reduced tissue thyroid level and a reduced ability to convert T4 to the active form of thyroid T3. He also found that rT3 is not the inert thyroid form once thought. He said high levels of it are also a marker for Hypothyroidism. He was seeing patients who had gastric bypass surgery, gaining all of their weight back even though they were on a supervised 800 calorie diet per day. They were found to be both leptin resistant and had low thyroid tissue levels. For these leptin resistant unfortunate individuals, all of my previous nutritional advice may not be sufficient. However, I would suggest that they get on line and investigates Dr. Ken Holtorf's article on this subject.

Thus, for most people, to stay within a healthy and fit bodyweight range does one have to watch what they eat forever? Well, the common sense answer to that is **OF COURSE THEY DO!** Now it is true that we are constantly being subliminally bombarded with suspect and sometimes deceptive food advertisements. We must exercise some self-control to avoid them. Finally, expert psychologists today recommend, when dieting one should not eliminate all of his favorites, but rather just eat the less nutritious foods **very** infrequently.

CHAPTER EIGHTEEN

Functional Medicine

You may be shaking your head saying to yourself, "Where do I start with this getting healthy, I have high blood pressure, adult onset diabetes and am overweight," or, "I have hormonal problems etc.?" Those patients with chronic neck and back pain usually ask what they can do about a certain specific problem found with their last blood work results. I explain that when interpreting blood work, I use "functional ranges" since I am a certified functional medicine practitioner.

Functional medicine is a non-traditional approach to managing chronic conditions by treating each patient individually. No two patients are metabolically identical; therefore, they cannot be treated in the same way. Functional medicine seeks first to identify and find the root cause of a problem while viewing the body as one integrated system. This is often the perfect fit for those who have not obtained needed answers through traditional medicine.

These functional ranges I use are not the same used by the medical profession, and are mainly used by such practitioners as naturopathic doctors, nutritionists and chiropractors specializing in nutrition and many others. Based on intensive research, functional ranges have been set to monitor good health before disease or pathology develops. Most lab tests come with ranges that medical doctor use; these ranges are really pathological ones which are good for diagnosing diseases but do very little as a measuring stick for ideal health. These pathological ranges were formulated by averaging all of the blood test results people had over many years. Obviously, many of these people are in poor health. Furthermore, if their test results are in the high normal "pathological" range, they have had the problem for a long time. Many positive lab findings could have been reversed before they became pathological by using functional ranges. Thus most of these people will now need to take medications to keep them in the "normal" range which was inaccurately determined?

Functional medicine also uses specific lab tests to find the true cause of the patient's current health problem. We call functional medicine "patient specific" care; it addresses the biochemical individuality of each of us. In other words, you cannot use the same cook book approach to every patient's symptoms. Traditional medicine on the other hand, along with many alternative medical doctors and chiropractors use "disease specific" care. They usually give the same drug or supplement to everyone with similar symptoms. This is the "throw as much mud on the wall and some will stick" approach. Keep in mind however; the chronic patients who cannot seem to get better have already been treated this way.

Let me give you some examples of functional versus pathological ranges. I previously mentioned the fact that many people are autoimmune; their bodies are attacking themselves. I must re-introduce and stress the importance of TSH or thyroid stimulating hormone because autoimmune thyroid disease is the most common autoimmune condition. Pathological ranges for TSH are anywhere from .35-5.5 MIU/L or so, but the most commonly used functional ranges TSH, are between 1.8-3.0 MIU/L.

More and more alternative doctors today are shocked by the plethora of hypothyroid sufferers with "normal test results" exhibiting terrible symptoms. These patients were told by medical doctors, "it is all in your head". The blood work of most female patient's I have been seeing, displayed high TSH readings, 4 or 5 MIU/L which is within the medical interpretation of "normal range". These women's complaints are the symptoms of a sluggish thyroid or hypothyroidism. When I ask them if they were tested for thyroid antibodies the answer is usually no, because the medical profession does not really treat autoimmune thyroid also known as Hashimotos.

The medical doctor will usually just prescribe prednisone when a flare up of Hashimotos occurs, and tell these patients "There is nothing else you can do for it". Functional medicine practitioners beg to differ. I tell patients all of the time that the molecular structure of the thyroid and gluten is almost identical. Anytime they eat foods containing gluten, their bodies attack the thyroid. I also explain that they **MUST** go gluten free. According to Dr. O'Bryan, thyroid antibodies are predictive for onset of Hashimotos within 7 years. Furthermore, researchers found that one of the most severe consequences of poorly managed Hashimotos is brain degeneration. Shockingly, researchers also have found that Hashimotos patients run a HUGE risk of developing Parkinson's or Alzheimer's disease.

Yet, many patients we send for thyroid anti-body testing come back negative. Why would this be? Remember when I talked about the TH1 and TH2 components of the immune system? These autoimmune thyroid patients have an imbalance in their TH1 and TH2 cells in which the TH2 system is often depressed not making enough anti-bodies to measure on a blood test. Furthermore, gluten in the diet and stressful events such as pregnancy can also alter the TH1 and TH2 balance.

My daughter Alexis, at age 17, was diagnosed with this autoimmune disorder. After years of her struggling with inconsistent symptoms of abdominal pain and fatigue, and no answers, I sent her to be tested for the thyroid peroxidase and anti-thyroglobulin antibodies. Both were present in high numbers and I was able to diagnose her with Hashimotos. Ironic, medical doctors told us years earlier during frequent visits to the emergency room, "It is not a matter of if she'll have a thyroid disorder; it's a matter of when." Because they had not tested her for an autoimmune disorder, her symptoms continued to worsen with age until the summer after she graduated from high school, when I joined the Johnson Group and realized the importance of the gluten free/autoimmune connection. A medical doctor would have put her on synthroid, synthetic thyroid medication, and she would have gone about living, slowly deteriorating internally, since that drug would not have gotten to the root of the problem. Fortunately, she went completely gluten free, and three years later, is still gluten free with NO symptoms.

Other blood markers for autoimmune thyroid include triglycerides of less than 75mg/Dl. The functional range is 75-100 mg/Dl and the medical range is less than 150mg/Dl. Another marker is higher HDLs greater than 70 mg/Dl. The functional range for HDLs is 55-100 mg/Dl and the medical range is equal to or greater than 46mg/Dl. Still another marker is cholesterol less than 150 mg/dl. These three findings, for example, indicate oxidative stress from free radicals, resulting from the S.A.D. **Remember cholesterol is one of the body's most potent antioxidants**. Functional ranges for cholesterol are 150-200 mg/Dl and the medical range is 125-200mg/DL. There may also be high homocysteine levels greater than 7umol/L. Functional ranges should be less than 7umol/L. Medical ranges are from 5.4-11.9 umol/L. Homocysteine is a toxic amino acid which can damage the lining of the arteries. High homocysteine means that the necessary methylation of the cells is not working properly leaving the patient at risk for disease. Finally, we can look at high sensitive C-reactive protein which optimally should be 0-3mg/L; anything greater is abnormal indicating inflammation.

When looking at Type II diabetes, we must consider both blood glucose and hemoglobin A1C functional ranges. Functional ranges for glucose are between 85-99 mg/Dl while normal medical range is between 90-120mg/Dl. The functional range for Hemoglobin A1C is 4.8-5.6% and the medical range here is less than 7.6%. Medical doctors only test the patient for this if he is diabetic or pre-diabetic, close to the 120mg/Dl levels.

This test is used to assess long-term glucose control especially in insulin dependent diabetes. However, some of the blood glucose and hemoglobin, the major component in the red blood cell functioning to transport oxygen in the blood, mix together forming an irreversible "glycohemoglobin" protein bond. The amount found in the red blood cell is the amount available in the blood. This functional range, along with the blood glucose, will pick up pre-diabetes. I remember my mother telling me that she asked her doctor to test her for hemoglobin A1C and he answered that it is only for diabetics. You may have to argue for this test from with your doctor.

I think by now you realize that functional medicine practitioners try to discover any imbalance in the systems as quickly as possible before a disease can occur. Some patients will read this and scratch their heads and wonder why their endocrinologists do not "know this" or find this to be true. I actually found an article titled, "Why Doesn't My Endocrinologist Know ALL of This?", written by Kent Holtorf MD and on the website of the National Academy of Hypothyroidism. The web address is http://nahypothyroidism.org. It is readily available. I have to thank whoever put this on the forum so I could discover it. Basically, the article explains that an overwhelming majority of physicians, endocrinologists, internists, family practitioners, and rheumatologists, do not read medical journals. He claims that when asked, most doctors say they read them. In reality, however, they do not always have the time and are too busy running their practices. Thus, most of them practice what they learned in school and use the treatment protocols of their medical societies, such as the American Association of Clinical Endocrinologists, for example, to direct treatment decisions. This practice has been graded by a number of organizations including the World Health Organization. Their denunciation of these practices is alarming and needs a direct quote: "All grading systems place consensus statements and expert opinion by respected authorities (societies) as the poorest level of evidence, because historically they have failed to adopt new concepts and treatments based on new knowledge or new-found understanding demonstrated in the medical literature."

The Endocrine Society, the American Association of Clinical Endocrinologists, and the American Thyroid Association also have a long history of not adopting new guidelines when new research contradicts their existing recommendations. That sounds a lot like the drug industry's influence. The author, Dr. Holtorf, sites an example in which these societies ruled out any thyroid abnormalities because the TSH range was normal despite "massive amounts of literature that demonstrates this not to be the case." These societies also disagreed with doctors endorsing T4 replacement only as adequate for patient health. The evaluating organizations felt, that doctors who only go by these blood test levels and ignore the clinical aspects of a patient are not practicing "evidence- based medicine." They continue to say these doctors are "adequate as lab technicians, but as doctors and clinicians they fall short." Remember there are several thyroid tests in order for a proper evaluation of the thyroid. Just evaluating TSH is not enough. The body will make 94% of thyroid hormone as T4, the inactive form, and only 7% as T3, the active form. This means it must convert the majority of T4 to T3 in you liver and gastrointestinal tract. Just prescribing a patient T4, synthroid without addressing and supporting the organs that have to convert it does not make sense. There must be a reason that the body is not converting it to T3 in the first place.

Now to be honest with you, my functional medicine patient's testing recommendations are different now than before. In other words, I used to order a complete metabolic blood panel, Cyrex panels 1-4, an

Adrenal Stress Index, and a Metametrix stool microbial panel on every patient with thyroid complaints. These test results would give me a great amount of information on assessing the patients' health, but for the most part were not covered by insurance. The initial testing cost about $2500 not to mention any re-tests three months later to assess progress. Over the years, I have seen many patients who did the tests I ordered and then came back to my office for a consultation not pleased with my diagnosis and treatment plan; so they went to a medical practitioner who told the ex-patient what they wanted to hear: "That chiropractor does not know what he is taking about; your thyroid is within the normal range. There is nothing wrong with you. Eat what you want." Therefore, as their health continued to deteriorate they took medications to relieve their symptoms. So many times people are told that there is nothing that can be done for their condition. Often times, the treatment I recommended for these patients would have drastically improved their lifestyle. This meant giving up foods containing dairy, soy, gluten and sugar, for example. Regrettably, many were not willing make the necessary sacrifices required for this long term, lifestyle change. **I have found that it does not always matter what the test results show if you are not willing to make certain changes.**

Currently, I have modified my treatment plans. When prospective patients come into my office looking for answers on how to treat their poor health, for example, they have complaints or symptoms, I offer some options. I can treat them with functional medicine, putting on my detective hat and order the minimal testing to provide the answers to address their complaint. I also can treat these patients with QRA, NanoSRT sensitivity reduction, diet counseling, and nutritional lifestyle changes for total health. I try to totally balance the body systems which will address and their hopefully remedy their original complaint.

Many chronically ill patients usually have already gone to medical doctors, had a ton of testing done, and did not improve with conventional medical care. Doctors never ordered the correct test(s) in order to find the cause of their problem. There are many functional medicine tests that I order which are unknown to Medical doctors. If these doctors do not except the functional medicine rationale, why should anyone think they will know anything about our less popular, diagnostic tests? For example, a Red blood cell (RBC) Mineral Test is used to discover what is happening in the cell, not in the serum outside of the cells. For instance, you could have "normal" serum magnesium levels according to your traditional medical blood test results, but have very low cellular magnesium according to the RBC Mineral Test. **This predicament is abnormal and puts your heart at high risk for an arrhythmia and possibly a heart attack.** Remember, adrenaline holds magnesium in the blood; therefore I also look to the adrenal glands when there is an arrhythmia and a magnesium deficiency. Think about this; if you have low cellular magnesium, your body will try to compensate by increasing your serum magnesium. If it is not in the cell, it cannot help the body. How accurate then is just a CBC blood test to evaluate minerals? It is, in fact, inaccurate. Another test most people never heard of is a Cardio Ion test that looks at what nutrition your body lacks or what nutrition is not being converted to energy from the foods you are eating. The American Heart Association stated that one out of three Americans has some sort of cardiovascular disease. The Cardio Ion test measures the risk factors for cardiovascular disease such as: homocysteine, fibrinogen, CoQ-10, fatty acid imbalances, C-reactive protein, and insulin, all which can be positively altered by improving nutrition. These are just a few examples of some of the less popular but necessary tests a functional practitioner may order.

Let me give you an example of one of my patients who initially came to the office for back pain. While I was treating the pain one day, he informed me that he also suffered from chronic high blood pressure not managed apparently even by high doses of high blood pressure medication. He said even high doses of blood pressure medication did not work. **Remember, high blood pressure is a sign of metabolic imbalance and not a disease.** In addition to the original paperwork, I gave him a 23 page comprehensive medical questionnaire to fill out. His had checked for: night sweats, dark circles under his eyes, hemorrhoids, bizarre dreams, sensitivity to car exhaust, and that he was a recovered alcoholic. These boxes checked all indicate severe liver stress/toxicity. Based on these findings and his other case information, I needed to rule out the following: a bacterial pathogen, heavy metal toxicity, and nutritional deficiencies- namely minerals. I also had to evaluate his liver function, fatty acid metabolism, and antioxidant status. I ran a complete blood count and metabolic panel. His blood test showed abnormal levels of uric acid, calcium, phosphorous, Bun, RBCs, HCT, and Hg on the function scale; this all indicated heavy metal toxicity. An advanced test, called a toxic metal blood test, also showed that his lead levels were off the charts. Chronic Lead and mercury exposure, even at lower levels can produce hypertension or high blood pressure. A little more digging and I found that he was a painter many years ago when paint was, you guessed it, lead based. Thus the answer was a treatment plan which incorporated a heavy metal detoxification process in addition to his blood pressure medicine. The patient's blood pressure then started to normalize on his re-evaluation visit 30 days later and returned to normal within 60 days. I usually do not expect these patients to drastically change their lifestyle, diet etc., since they just want the symptoms or their condition to improve. Some, however, will go further with treatment for total health and surprise me. The total health of patients, my main goal, is to achieve metabolic and neurological balance. I described earlier how I treat neurologically. To address them metabolically, I initially have them keep a food journal so that we both know everything they have eaten in the last month or so. I also recommend the NanoSRT procedure to treat sensitivities and QRA, which uses muscle testing, to see what nutritional supplements they may need. Any blood, urine and stool sample testing to assess their general health is optional. There are instances in which a patient has some abnormal functional ranges on blood work they brought along; I ordered a follow up study a few months later after treatment for comparison. As I just stated, when you balance the body this way, hopefully, all of the symptoms and complaints go away. Even some patients who have no complaints still want the tests proving results in black and white. The patient who chooses this type of care is one who is more concerned about health than just about symptoms.

So to summarize, when prospective patients come to my office with musculoskeletal problems, neck and back pains, as most do, I recommend chiropractic service, laser, traction, atm, and/or the other modalities I described earlier. If they mention any other complaints such as high blood pressure, indigestion, reflux, fatigue etc... I will always suggest blood work and offer them natural treatment with functional medicine a long with their family doctor's. I gladly welcome those who just want to relieve of their symptoms naturally, along with those who want to become healthier and really change their lifestyles. Once the patient's health concerns have improved and the pain has lessened by using functional medicine, I recommend QRA and "grocery list" maintenance supplements, for those who want to maintain a more overall healthy lifestyle.

CHAPTER NINETEEN

Talking the Walk and Walking the Talk

In this chapter I will explain my particular life regimen. This includes nutrition, exercise, and the rationale behind them. I will try to give my rational as I go along. The previous sections of the book contain information based on research, facts, professional study, work experience and continual investigation. In the last two chapters I am going to interject much of my own opinion based on my 34 years of weight training and nutritional experience.

Monday through Friday I begin my day with core exercises; 5 twenty five rep sets of abdominal exercises and 2 twenty five rep sets of spinal erector exercises each day rotating individual exercises. On at Monday, Wednesday, and Friday, at 5am I go to Gold's gym where I do 40 minutes of weight training followed by twenty minutes of cardio. I do legs one day, chest and triceps the next, and back and biceps last. Of course eventually I rotate the workout so that my body never gets used to one exercise regimen. On Tuesday and Thursday, I do a kettle bell workout at home, focusing on the shoulders and external rotators more on Thursday.

Spinal erector extension exercises are extremely important and need explanation. Because most people are familiar with abdominal exercises such as crunches and sit-ups, I will not describe them. My goal is to exercise the complete abdominal area, upper, lower, and transverse using a variety of exercises.

More importantly, most people's daily life's activities usually involve some sort of forward flexion of the torso, meaning a person is bent over forward at the waist. The seated position is really like bending forward. Not many jobs or activities involve bending backwards, or extension at the waist, except for drywall installers or painters, for

233

example. This repetitive forward flexion without extension is the reason almost everyone on the planet develops lower back pain at some time or another. Therefore, we should all be doing some low back extension exercises on a daily basis or at least three times per week. Let me describe a few of the extension exercises I do, using a swiss ball for a couple of them; it is a large rubber ball that you pump up with air on which you perform various exercises and yoga moves. These balls come in various sizes; I use a medium sized one about two feet tall. In one extension exercise I lie on my stomach on the swiss ball so that my upper body is unsupported; I am balancing on the ball like a teeter totter. I then lower my upper body to the ground and return to the starting position, using my toes to steady myself during this exercise. You can have your arms at your sides or hold them out in front of you or even grip some dumbbells to make this more challenging. Another exercise with the swiss ball is a cross crawl pattern. While lying on my stomach, instead of just moving my torso up and down, I will extend my left arm out in front of me while at the same time lifting my right leg up. Then I will lower both my left arm and right leg only to raise the right arm with my left leg. When both arms and legs have been raised and lowered, that is one repetition. I perform one set of twenty five repetitions. This is great for core stabilization since you must be able to balance on the swiss ball the whole time. This cross crawl can also be a great brain exercise to correct imbalance between the two firing sides of the brain. I also do an exercise, lying on my stomach on the floor with my hands at my sides. I then lift my arms out in front of me as if I were flying and hold this position five to ten seconds before lowering them. This will really warm up the spinal erector muscles; three to five repetitions are sufficient. A variation of this is where you also raise your legs up a few inches off the floor while you raise your arms out in front of you. Do not try this for the first time while experiencing low back following an injury.

On Tuesdays and Thursdays I try to work different muscles in a different way than traditional weights do, an example of cross fit; you may have heard of it. A few examples of cross fit exercises would be when one flips over a huge truck tire, drags an anchor, or carries heavy weights in each hand while trying to walk as quickly as possible. Currently, on Thursday, I also do a group of external rotation muscle exercises consisting of rubber tubing and dumbbells which develop the muscles of the shoulder that make up the rotator cuff. I do four or five exercises in succession with no rest to really fatigue these muscles. Moreover, working these muscles will immensely help your shoulders to avoid future problems. I have seen many sedentary patients over the years who just reached in the back seat of the car for something or at home in bed for their alarm clock only to hear the pop of the rotator cuff followed by an excruciating pain. Moreover there are the serious weight lifters who injure their shoulders because they neglected to exercise this important, external rotator muscle group. As a result they look "Neanderthal like", meaning their head is jutting forward and their shoulders are rolling in. In the course of a day we are constantly engaged in activities in which we are pushing forward and adducting our arms in a hugging motion such as with reaching for a can or turning a steering wheel. We also need to exercise the external rotators of the shoulder and upper back more in order to enable us to keep our head straight and shoulders back because gravity will succeed, otherwise, pushing the head and shoulders forward to such an extent it looks as though a person is sniffing the ground. A larger busted woman really needs to exercise these muscles due to the fact that they carry permanent weight on the front of them, unbalancing the body. Breast tissue, if unopposed by counter muscles in the upper back and external rotators, will force your upper body forward and your shoulders to roll in and also often result in chronic back pain. *Exercising your external rotator shoulder muscles can REALLY save you from future SHOULDER AND POSTURAL problems.*

After the shoulder workout, I stand on the vibration plate for ten minutes. On the vibe plate I am constantly standing on one leg and contracting my core; this forces me to contract those muscles while being shaken and to use a lot of stabilizer muscles not normally used.

On Monday and Thursday I also do a ten to fifteen minute yoga type stretch, after my workout, incorporating such positions as the downward facing dog, extended triangle, and plank pose. Maintaining some flexibility as we age is necessary; without it you will simply lose muscle and joint function that much sooner. Generally, I do not do formal exercise on the weekends, but then I really do not sit still much either. Becky and I often walk the dog on weekends when the weather is nice. Living in a house built in 1850 on 2 1/3 acres, I have a continual supply of house and garden chores. The reason for continual movement is to keep the joints nourished. When we just sit around the joints get stiff just like a door's hinges needing oil or like the Tin man in the Wizard of Oz. **There is no doubt that resistance training is the most important of all exercises. You have to use the muscle or you will lose the muscle and consequently the function that those muscles control. It does not matter how old you are; there are types of resistance training one can do at any age**. The resistance bands, for example, are great. Many come in a portable pulley system that you just attach to your door like the one I bought my father recently, and so I know many kinds are available. There is also something called "The Easy Shaper Pro" which uses elastic cords you can buy on line. If you want to be able to take care of yourself as you age and not be dependent on others, you must maintain normal muscle function. I tell patients that the important reason for this is not merely a matter of appearance but function. Being able to walk to the refrigerator and bathroom without a cane or walker could become very difficult for many of you reading this if YOU DO NOT BEGIN AN EXERCISE ROUTINE AND STICK TO IT. There is no tomorrow either; do not keep putting it off. The buck stops here. Okay, enough of the Vince Lombardi pep talk. You get the idea of how important exercise and movements are to our continually aging bodies.

All animals instinctively know they need activity or exercise. Look at your domestic animals that actually are fully functional almost up until the day they die; unless we interfere with Mother Nature's natural selection process of dying. When an animal is lying around and not able to move, his whole body shuts down quickly. Think of us as smart animals whenever you do not feel like exercising.

On M-W-F, I also do cardio at the gym alternating machines such as the treadmill, the elliptical, Cyrex, and the recumbent bike. I vary the training so the heart, lungs, and all muscles involved are constantly guessing; again, the same goes for the weight training.

I cannot believe how much time people spend in the gym doing a workout, sitting around on equipment for minutes at a time between exercises. This is really wasting time and accomplishing nothing. The key to building lean muscle is to keep your weight training workouts to about 40 minutes. I do supersets and giant sets going from one exercise to another without much rest so I can get a lot done in a short time. Otherwise the stress hormone, cortisol, is secreted, having a catabolic or tissue breakdown effect on muscle. To build a healthy, strong, and leaner muscular body, we need an anabolic or tissue building effect on muscle. If you are trying to get lean and muscular, you must work out with resistance or weights for about 40 minutes and do cardio for 20-30 minutes afterwards. This is because any glycogen you have in the liver and muscle will be burned after 30-40 minutes or so and then you start to burn fat. Thus by the end of your resistance workout, you should have depleted the sugar in your muscles and liver and are now burning fat. Now it is true that you do not have to do any exercise at all- and based on what you eat, or do not eat, you can lose all the weight you need to. But there is a catch in losing weight without exercising; **you will actually lose a lot of**

muscle along with the fat. This will make your resting metabolism even slower in the long run. **Exercise will definitely minimize any muscle loss that would occur with the fat loss.**

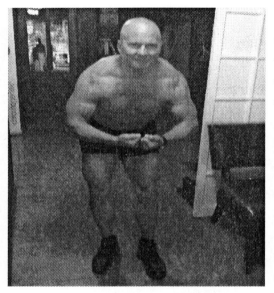

Figure 1: Me "Walking The Talk" 9/24/13

I will now discuss my current diet in some detail. After waking up on weekdays, I was eating a slice of gluten free bread with almond or cashew butter but have since stopped, I realizing that bread defeats the purpose when trying to achieve more muscularity. Keep in mind if eat bread, even gluten free and non-GMO has too many processed ingredients unless you bake it from scratch. It is very hard to bake gluten free bread from scratch however, or even a mix, and achieve the right consistency; it usually comes out like cake and not something you can easily slice for sandwiches. Remember, we should strive to eat most foods that are limited to a few ingredients. Thus, I do not eat bread on a regular basis but only occasionally. If you want to eat the gluten free bread then go right ahead. The Paleo websites offers many grain free substitutes. Becky and I just had coconut/tapioca flour dinner rolls from a www.paleospirit.com recipe this past Thanksgiving. They were delicious right out of the oven spread with butter and tasted better than the regular rolls sold. Another recipe we tried was Paleo cauliflower garlic bread made with eggs and cheese but no flour. I know this sounds incredible but it has the consistency of bread! If you google Paleo cauliflower garlic bread, you will find several Paleo sites that have this recipe among other good ones.

My post workout meal is usually a green shake that I drink right at the end of my workout. I also drink a whole bottle of water during the workout to ensure proper hydration. When I get home, I make a bowl of gluten free oatmeal. There is a big controversy over oatmeal and whether it is contaminated by wheat since it may be made in the same facility. Therefore the brands I use are from the organic gluten free section of either Wegmans or Giant Foods grocery, either "Eco-planet" or "Glutenfreeda." To the oatmeal I add cinnamon, blueberries, coconut milk and one teaspoon of Canadian golden honey with half of teaspoon of Camellia pollen FX, both PRL products for liver health. Incidentally, this honey is the best tasting I have ever eaten. Because grains do turn to sugar so quickly, I only eat oatmeal on my most strenuous workout days. The body needs nourishment within two hours preferably immediately post workout because the muscle cells are more receptive to proteins and sugars to replenish the glycogen you just burned off. On my lighter workout days and on weekends, when I do not lift any weights, I eat a three-egg omelet for breakfast with a potato browned in olive oil and broccoli. Sometimes I add some seasoned ground chicken or turkey for more protein.

I began drinking green shakes, a concoction that I devised, on the suggestion of a good friend. We both had chiropractic offices in the same building from 1995-1997 in Camp Hill. I bought a book called *"Green for Life"* by Victoria Boutenko that his wife found fascinating. The author stated that people with chronic diseases were regaining their health by giving up processed foods and drinking these green shakes daily. Although, I always realized the importance of the leafy green veggies, I neglected to eat them because most of the greens are difficult to chew raw. Gorillas actually chew them for an hour working them into a paste. Yuk. Cooking them is also not as beneficial since it destroys many of the nutritive enzymes. Becky and I sauté greens about once per week in olive oil, but I am still drinking the green shakes in the morning. Thus when I read the Green for life book it was as if a bell rang in my head. I decided I could drink a good serving of leafy greens and easily get this huge dose of anti-oxidants. Leafy greens are among the best foods for our bodies, yet probably the most neglected. Most Americans never eat them. Peas and corn are the vegetables usually eaten on a regular basis by most people in this country. The *"Green for Life"* book gives a lot of examples of how to camouflage the sometimes bitter taste of greens that turn most people away. Since the taste is not a main concern for me, I cautious not to add too much fruit to make them palatable. **You should try to eat twice the amount of green leafy vegetables as fruits due to the high sugar content of fruit.** Select mostly fruits with a stone or a pit; these contain the lowest glycemic indexes.

Years ago, I remember talking to my friend John when he owned the Gold's Gym in town that I currently train. I said, "John, why don't you offer a green protein shake so that people can get the greens in their system along with the regular protein?" He unfortunately replied, "Because you and I would be the only ones drinking them, brother." Then it hit me that the public really tends to put too much emphasis on taste; most care a lot about taste but it seems to be at the expense of health.

A "protein shake" in the morning seems to be the rave right now. Everybody is asking me about protein shakes which I have been drinking for as long as I have been weight training. However, as I stated earlier, I started adding the greens in 1996. Many people ask how much protein they should consume for both weight loss and overall general health. I recently read an important article by Douglas Anderson DC, CCN (certified clinical nutritionist) titled "Protein and Weight Loss." He talks reveals how competitive the fitness and nutrition industry are and how they are multi-billion dollar businesses that market of exercise equipment, exercise plans, and supplements. His summation must be quoted: "The information Age we live in produces a constant stream of new research that is rapidly disseminated, selectively edited, commonly misinterpreted and excessively extrapolated- usually for secondary financial gain." This also holds so true for Big Pharma with drug sales. He follows it with, "The biochemical and physiological diversity of people means there is more than one path to the top of the weight loss mountain." When people asked him about how many grams of protein per day to consume, he answered, "Just the right amount for building lean muscle and losing fat that keeps your hunger at bay". This amount of course, also depends on your age, sex, activity level, and genetics. Certainly, Dr. Anderson's answer is the best one I have heard to date. People who gained weight recently should start keeping a log of what they are eating each day so that they know how many grams of protein they are consuming. My buddy Dave, who owned a gym for twenty-five years, is like a walking nutrition almanac. After choosing a day's menu, he knows exactly how much protein and how many calories he will eat in a day and divides it out by six or seven small meals; that is his formula. I am not suggesting anybody has to follow Dave's precise formula, but if you are overweight, consider increasing protein intake; you may lose more unwanted fat and build more lean muscle. Protein usually satisfies most peoples hunger to a greater degree than carbohydrates and even fats and also requires more calories to process or metabolize than either of them. Thus your metabolic rate can be increased for up to 10-12 hours after eating any proteins. Remember, however, **most people have low stomach acid, and that is exactly what you need to absorb protein.** For strength training athletes, Dr. Anderson suggests 1.2-1.4 grams of protein per kilogram of bodyweight (2.2 pounds). For most women it would be about .8 grams, and for most men it would be about 1 gram. In my opinion, for those who work out regularly should have 1 gram per pound of bodyweight. I try to take 1 gram per pound of bodyweight; you can experiment. However, excess protein is broken down to ammonia and then further to urea and uric acid to be secreted in the urine. Therefore, since there is controversy concerning how processing any extra protein the body does not need will tax the kidneys, it is important to determine just how much your body needs.

The green shake I drink immediately after my workout includes 30-40 grams of whey protein. Research shows that your body can only metabolize or process 30-40 grams of protein per hour to build muscle. I try to get it from a source that has no fillers, artificial sweeteners, and no soy. PRL has whey protein and the "Jay Robb" brand does also. Into the shake go one or two big leaves of Swiss chard, kale, collards, or two tablespoons of Bragg's Apple Cider vinegar to prevent any oxalate stones forming from the collards especially, a banana, and a tablespoon of Chia seeds, plant based omega three fatty acids which really help with overall body inflammation. Those are the ingredients of my morning protein shake, if you have a lot of problems with dairy, there is a pea protein and a beef protein available at "Designs for health" and www.designsfor health.com. Using a vitamix, I make five days' worth of green shakes on Sunday for the upcoming week and refrigerate them in five glass bottles.

My first supplement of the day "so to speak" is taken after I turn the morning shower off, by moisturizing with organic unrefined coconut oil, applying it all over face and body. Remember, breathing it in, rubbing it in, eating and drinking something are all methods of getting nutrients into your body. A few days a week, I also use coconut oil in the shower for "oil pulling" to get help the body get rid of toxins. I just swish a teaspoon or so around in my mouth for the duration of the shower and then just spit it out. I think it helps with the silver fillings I have until I can get them removed.

My supplements for breakfast are as follows: ½ teaspoon of liquid *Green Tea ND*, ½ teaspoon of *Max Stress B*, 3-6 drops of *Vit D3-* depending on season and sun exposure, and one ounce of Aloe pro mixed in a few ounces of water. A couple times per year, I add ½ teaspoon of both *gallbladder ND* and *Liver ND* to support and detox both of them. I also add a teaspoon of *Essential Fatty Acids,* which contain borage, sesame, evening primrose oil, and black currant oil, together known as prostaglandin series one. They, like the omega 3s or prostaglandin series 3, are used for their anti-inflammatory effects. For variety, I alternate the Essential fatty acids liquid with 2-3 *DHA* capsules daily for three successive months. Two capsules of *HCL*, one *Digest*, one *Activator*, in addition to one *NZ-Red Velvet Deer Antler* capsule, and three *Coral Legend Plus* capsules for minerals, to keep the pH in the 6.4-7.0 range, are the final breakfast supplements.

At 10:15 am I eat a snack of mixed nuts excluding peanuts. Lunch is usually fish or ground chicken or estrogen free turkey that Becky spiced up with onions, peppers, garlic, etc., accompanied by a sweet potato. Veggies are usually broccoli or green beans, vegetable soup, some guacamole or hummus with organic non GMO rice flour tortilla chips we made and cooked in coconut oil. Be careful of the junk oils like safflower, canola, or sunflower, on the tortilla chips label. Finally, I have an apple with organic almond, sesame, or cashew butter on it. I always drink water and sometimes herbal tea. Sometimes for variety, I choose grass fed beef or buffalo as a protein source.

My supplements for lunch are: *HCL*, *HCL Activator*, *Premier Digest*, *DHA*, and two *IP6* capsules; in addition I also take one *Premier testosterone* capsule. I ALWAYS eat vegetables at lunch; however, if I am out somewhere vegetables are not available; I add to two *Premier Greens* capsules.

For a snack, three days a week or so, I have an organic protein bar from PRL around 3pm., mostly for convenience, a quick and easy way to get the 22 grams of protein and 300 calories to sustain me while I am seeing patients until dinner time. On other days I may eat coconut yogurt, grass fed beef jerky, a homemade nut bar, or Paleo pancakes.

At dinner time, I usually eat some type of organic chicken breast, from a variety of recipes, combined with long grain brown rice, broccoli or green beans, and a greens salad. We also eat many kinds of casseroles with cabbage and spinach, artichokes, zucchini, Brussels sprouts, and tomatoes. Sometimes, we use gluten free spaghetti from rice flour, or spaghetti squash with turkey meatballs and Bove's organic sugar free tomato sauce.

There are many grain free substitutes, from yet another Paleo website: www.paleOmg.com, for rice that I will also eat to mix it up. Again for variety we may eat fish or grass fed beef burgers, or turkey meat loaf. My supplements here are the same as at lunch time.

Speaking of beef, patients often ask me about vegetarianism and its offshoots. There are vegans who eat dairy and others who will not eat dairy but will eat poultry, known as pollotarians; those vegetarians who eat fish are called pescatarians. Then there are flexitarians who usually eat no meat, but once in a while their diet does include meat and fish? They also eat more whole grains, legumes, fresh fruits and veggies thus claiming to have "flexibility" in their healthy lifestyle pursuits. This diet is acceptable as long as the grains contain no gluten. I have concerns about the lack of Vitamin A and Vitamin D in both the non-meat and non-dairy vegetarians' diets. Lack of sun and the use of sunscreen limited the Vit D available from this source. And the best food sources for Vit D and Vit A are animal products such as fish, butter and liver as well as non- animal sources such as olive oil for Vit A and mushrooms for Vit D. The precursor to vitamin A, beta carotene, can be obtained from fruits and vegetables but must be converted; those with a sluggish thyroid, diabetes, and celiac disease, however, have a much harder time converting it Vit A.

Now many vegetarians will say that red meat consumption leads to general inflammation and avoid it. This is partially true because most cows are fed not the necessary grass, but soybeans and corn, the causes of this inflammation. Since we do not consume the entire animal with its organs as our ancestors did, the body will produce high amounts of homocysteine, the toxic amino acid I described earlier. And both highly processed carbohydrates as well as stress deplete the necessary Vitamin B supply needed to convert the homocysteine to cysteine so it can be eliminated from the body. If, however, you eat grass fed beef and do not ingest highly processed carbohydrates and are not under extreme amounts of stress the beef causing inflammation dilemma does not occur.

I always snack at 9-9:30 pm. I usually have an organic rice cake and an apple with almond butter spread and also drink some coconut water. I try to check my first morning urine pH at least three times per week aiming for the 6.4-7.0 range.

Becky and I usually eat at a restaurant once or twice weekly. Dr. Marshall suggests taking along some *DHA* to counteract any fatty acids from the raunchy oils like canola used to cook pre-packaged foods because it is cheap. According to the Dr. Marshall, when a body is exposed to junk oils and good oils simultaneously, it chooses the good oils. If you are only exposed to the junk oils in a restaurant, that is what your body will absorb. Partially, but not fully hydrogenated, to deodorize it, canola oil does not have to be labeled as hydrogenated, a deceptive practice causing harm to many people. Keep in mind that this hydrogenated oil will then decrease the conversion of omega three fatty acids to DHA. Like me, if you are not eating out too often it is not problematic. However, for those of you who eat out almost every day, it may be beneficial to bring your own fatty acids. Premier *DHA* is from live source algae and is an excellent choice.

It is hard to be healthy and trim if you eat at restaurants often unless they are an organic or green one; unfortunately, there are not many of them around. Try to order chicken, fish, beef, vegetables, and salads, and not so much the calzones, pizzas, and strombolis. They do make gluten free substitutes but is still probably loaded with trans-fats and a lot of sugar. I know many people will use one day a week for a cheat day during which they may eat some junk, however, doing this more than once per week will defeat the purpose of maintaining a healthy weight and overall good health.

Becky and I are social drinkers; we often have a few drinks on weekends but not during the week. As by buddy Dave once said, "You have to live a little." Since all hard liquor is gluten-free as a result of the distilling process; theoretically, you can drink any hard liquor you choose. Many people, celiac sufferers for example, however will prefer to stick to the potato vodka, rum, and tequila which always were gluten free. I do not drink beer because as John so succinctly put it, "It will make you fat." Moreover, most beers except for a few, are wheat-based therefore, not gluten free. Certain wines containing a non-wheat clarifying agent are my choice when I infrequently drink wine.

This is my diet with supplements. As you are aware, nutritional research continues to provide information on newer and more efficient products such as PRL's reformulated *EFA*. Naturally, my diet and supplements will change to accommodate new findings.

Since we are constantly bombarded by all of the chemicals in the air, soil, water and GMO food, we should try to minimize the causes of inflammation and resulting, continuous free radical damage. Remember you cannot get all the nutrition you need from food alone.

I will discuss hygiene products beginning with toothpaste. The major brands are loaded with sodium lauryl sulfate therefore I use the

"Jason" brand. When many patients ask me about Tom's brands, I reply they were good until bought by Colgate who altered the natural formula. Most name brand anti-perspirants contain aluminum which plugs the sweat glands preventing secretion.

Anyone would surely agree that the idea of rubbing aluminum under the armpit is BAD NEWS. You can get easily find a crystal at a health food store which actually forms a layer of mineral salts over the skin, when rubbed under the arm, making it a poor environment for bacteria to thrive in and thus preventing any odor. Coconut oil can also be used under the arms as a deodorant. You can get "Jungle man" or "Jungle woman" deodorant on-line at Amazon. It is also being sold at certain health food stores. A google search will tell you which stores sell it. I currently use a combination of coconut oil and the Jungle man brand. This is the best natural deodorant to stop odor that both Becky and I have ever used.

PRL has a face cream with hyaluronic acid, one of the main ingredients in collagen, called *H.A. Repair Cream*. This hyaluronic acid prevents skin from wrinkling by giving it that plump appearance and also will give shape to the tissues around the eyes. Becky and I both use the cream on our eyes at night and also PRL's *Facial Cleanser* every morning; regular bar soap is garbage containing perfumes, chemicals, and other additives. Buy your soap at either the organic section of Giant or Wegmans or at a health food store. PRL also has glycerin based gentle hand soap. You can also find natural, "do it yourself" soap recipes.

This reminds me of how toxic perfumes can be. In fact, perfumes and colognes contain 85% petroleum. A large barrel with perfumes and colognes would be considered toxic and require someone in a hazmat suit to dispose of. Becky avoids perfume, and uses natural oils instead. Many people ask her what perfume she is wearing that smells so good. If you do use cologne or perfume, never put it on your skin; just spray it and walk into it, so that it only goes on your clothes. Try not to breathe in this toxic substance.

Shampoo, conditioners, and cosmetics also contain many of the same toxic chemicals. PRL has some natural alternatives, but of course you would not ask a bald man for his opinion on make-up and hair products now would you? Ha. "Wen" is supposedly natural, but one of the first ingredients is hydrolyzed wheat protein. There are several recipes online which use such ingredients as "coconut milk, apple cider vinegar, peppermint oil, tea tree oil, castle soap, baking soda, and olive oil." Yes, you are using many of the same ingredients you should also be eating! *Larenim Mineral* has a cosmetic line which you also find on the Internet. Remember, rubbing it in your skin is just like eating, drinking, or breathing it in- as far as toxic load build-up in your body is concerned.

Although summer has recently ended, as I write this, I must mention sunscreen. **A half an hour per day out in the sun is good for you.** If you need to apply sunscreen then make sure it is a brand without chemicals, such as Bert's Bees. Lying in a hot sun for hours wearing traditional chemical sunscreen seeping into your skin is definitely not wise. The sun's heat may facilitate and intensify the sunscreen's absorption of harmful chemicals.

I use PRL's all natural *Shave Gel* to shave my head and face every morning. It is an invisible gel you cannot even feel on your face or head; and provides a smooth shave with no irritation.

I must talk about electro-magnetic radiation from such electronics as cell phones and their towers. There is currently so much money made in the cell phone business; the negative adverse effects of EMF (electromagnetic fields) are downplayed. After attending a PRL/QRA seminar last year, I decided to block as many EMFs from cell phone towers as possible. I bought a twenty pound bag of *Dragonite*, a source of paramagnetic volcanic basalt minerals. This is a rock dust source which helps mineralize soil but it significantly blocks EMFs from getting through. By spreading the *Dragonite* out over the corners of my house and office, the two buildings were grounded. Some say this is an extreme measure, but the radiation is a real hazard; I feel better about having some protection from it. You can prove this protective effect with kinesiology by testing stronger in an area where there are no EMFs. Taking it one step further to actually block the EMF's coming from my cell phone, I bought PRL's *Q disc*, a small oval shaped, inch high, half inch wide disc that sticks to the back of the cell phone to block the cell phone radiation.

There are many other protective products out there you can investigate depending on how serious your health concerns are. Whatever your comfort zone, there are products to match it from organic sleep systems to lifestyle tools.

FINAL CHAPTER

Putting It All Together

To stay healthy and to live without problems that interfere with the normal daily activates, you must take care of the mind and as well as the body because mental stress is a killer. Each of us must have an outlet from the mental stress that accumulates during a normal day from work stress, problems with relatives, friends, etc. In addition to forms of meditation like yoga or spiritual healing that ameliorate stress levels, people suffering from mental stress should look into some type of physical activity like simple walking which is also a potent mental de-stressor that prevents the chance of adversely long term health.

Many of you reading this book may not have physical symptoms and, therefore, are not interested in going to any doctor for a checkup. On the other hand, however, some of you may be very curious about the state of your health. You can begin changing your health for the better by simply checking your first morning urine pH. Here we are looking for a range between 6.4 and 7.0. This urine pH evaluates your body's mineral content. If you are getting adequate minerals in your body, toxic heavy metals will not be able to bind to your cells. I also recommend the *HCL detox kit* and pancreatic enzymes with every meal because after you are 30 years old, the body does not have enough of either; less than thirty, you need the pink sea salt for your body can make its own HCL from the chloride in the sea salt. You may need pancreatic enzymes even when in your mid to upper-twenties if your diet is not adequate. Remember, the S.A.D. strips the essential fatty acids away leaving trans- fats and deaminated gluten added for long shelf life of many processed foods. If you suspect that your stomach acid is too high, you can do a burp test; drink a ¼ teaspoon of baking soda in an 8 ounce glass of water. You should burp within two minutes indicating your stomach acid is adequate. If it takes you longer or if you do not even burp at all, you have a condition called hypochlorohydria or low stomach acid. Other markers in your blood work can also indicate this lower level of stomach acid; for example, if your levels of total protein, phosphorous, carbon dioxide, globulin, MCV, MCH, and BUN are abnormal, it could indicate a stomach acid deficiency.

Just by doing these two things: Getting enough HCL and pancreatic enzymes along with keeping your pH between 6.4 and 7.0 will greatly impact your health in a positive way. In summary, the processed foods of today are so nutritionally inferior that our bodies have to use a lot of their energy to process them. Remember the liver must process these dietary toxins, requiring massive amounts of energy, with the result of insufficient enzymes left for normal digestion. Therefore, we must supplement our diet with enzymes.

Today many people, over 50% in fact, have chronic health problems because of bad nutrition. One of the reasons is that by cooking food you get rid of most of its nutritive value; it has been documented that up to 85% of a food's value is lost when cooked at high temperatures.

Patients often ask me which oils I cook with. Earlier, I talked about the benefits of coconut oil and recently about DHA and fish oil. The discussion about which oils should be ingested is confusing and often filled with misinformation and sometimes even filled with contradiction. A lot of this seems like a paradox or contradiction. I hope I made it easier for you to be comfortable with your choice of fatty acid oils. For example, I told you how healthy coconut oil is and went into detail.

To summarize, MONEY AND GREED is why, up until recently, it was categorically stated in all the media that all saturated fat is no good and causes heart attacks, etc. Remember the *"Cholesterol Con"*, written Dr. Anthony Colpo MD who discussed how saturated fat was vilified just like cholesterol. Anyone knowledgeable today in the field of nutrition endorses the benefits of coconut oil and coconut milk. Though coconut is saturated fat, it is saturated with hydrogen so there are no double bonds to break down when heated in cooking or when eaten and broken down by the body; coconut oil is very stable. On the other hand, polyunsaturated vegetable oils such as corn, soy, safflower, sunflower and canola, are the absolute worst oils to cook with because when heated, they OXIDIZE and cause free radical damage to our bodies; THEY ARE VERY UNSTABLE. These are all omega-6 oils, which are highly susceptible to heat damage because of their double bonds; they are not saturated with hydrogen molecules. Furthermore, just the way these junk oils are produced makes them unhealthy for our bodies whether you cook with them or not; thus, they go rancid in our bodies as soon as we ingest them. They are the reason left over foods taste worse than freshly cooked. If we look at oils with one double bond or mono saturated oils we can see that there is some "unsaturation." Since it is only one double bond, however, this is not too much; therefore, extra virgin olive oil is great for cooking. There is currently some controversy over whether to use high cooking temperatures with olive oil. Some say it is alright to cook on high, since the oil does not oxidize; others may insist that you should only use medium heat. If you get the extra virgin olive oil that is pure and unrefined, you get a high smoke point at 410 degrees while cooking with it; this is the high smoke point at which it breaks down when heated. You can investigate those claims on your own. In our house we cook with olive oil very frequently. If we then look at other poly unsaturated oils like omega-3 oils, such as flax oil, they contain three double bonds; THUS YOU DO NOT WANT TO HEAT OR COOK WITH THEM AT ALL. In fact they should be stored in the refrigerator or freezer and away from light whether in seed form or oil. **The omega-3s comprise a class of fatty acids that are classified as essential because the body cannot make them on its own.** As said many times, the health benefits, particularly their actions as anti-inflammatory agents and their anti-clotting tendency to reduce blood clots, cannot be denied. There is where the paradox lies. The omega 3 oils are also not stable enough for light and heat exposure nor are they manufactured by the body. However, numerous studies have proven that these essential oils provide many health benefits. The omega-6 fatty acids, although also essential, really work opposite omega-3 fatty acids by promoting inflammation and the tendency for clot formation. These are needed when you get injured and heal the body with inflammation; however, they are not needed nearly as often as the omega 3's ant-inflammatory effects are needed. One of the biggest nutritional problems is the use of the S.A.D. has negatively altered the proper omega-6 to omega-3 ratio causing widespread inflammation in the body. One might say the modern day diet has drastically changed over the last century; the cheaper and more plentiful omega-6s rule. As a consequence, the ratio has gone from an ideal 2:1 or 3:1 (omega-6s to omega-3s) to about 10:1 and even 20:1. Boy, that ratio certainly provides for a lot of inflammation and clotting tendencies. Can any of you reading this not agree that with this lopsided ratio come huge health risks? I hope you can now see how the stage is set for future problems such as stroke and cardiovascular issues. Think about the high blood work results concerning the levels of homocysteine, uric acid, C-reactive protein and fibrinogen, all inflammatory markers. To normalize the ratio, many nutritionists have been suggesting that people increase their dietary omega-3s from such foods as chia, flax, walnuts, and especially DHA and fish oils.

So there you have it; there is a lot to think about when it comes to fatty acids. A common sense approach would be to eat wild caught salmon a few times per week, take the EFA from PRL which has some unrefined cold pressed flaxseed oil, olive oil, sesame oil, and borage oil. In addition, take PRL's algae based DHA, moisturize with coconut oil and use coconut milk instead of cow's. As you should know by now, the algae based DHA is getting it right from the source, the fish not the middleman. Your body will then convert it to EPA as it needs it, if you are healthy. You should also grind up some chia seeds and put them in a green shake. Flaxseeds are phytoestrogens which mimic the effects of estrogen; plastics are also estrogenic and decrease your body's methylation process leading to chronic diseases.

High quality, organic cold pressed Flax oil, on the other hand, does not have any phytoestrogens. I no longer use Hemp seeds, although they contain 50-75% more protein per serving than flax or chia, because recent research established that they have very little fiber and only about 40% the omega-3 content of flax and chia. Moreover, their omega-6 content is very high; they will unfavorably alter the omega -6 to omega-3 fatty acid ratio.

Try to eat more raw uncooked food like fruits, and veggies. **The wheat in this country is slowly killing us all**. There is too much evidence suggesting the harmful effects of gluten. Investigate for yourself. Because so many people think that "a gluten free diet" is just another passing fad, I must take a final look at it disastrous effects on the body.

Becky recently handed me an excellent article titled, "This Is Your Gut on Gluten," by Anne Myers, M.D., founder and director of Austin Ultra Health, in which she describes what happens to the body when a person eats gluten.

After eating that morning bowl of Wheaties or Special K containing gluten, the enzyme tissue transglutaminase (tTG) is produced in your intestines and breaks the gluten down to gliadin and glutenin. These proteins travel through the intestines while the immune system in the gut, known as the "gut associated lymphoid tissue (GALT)," screens them for potentially harmful substances. If there is no sensitivity to gluten, the food gets absorbed. However, as Dr. Myers states, "In order to be drought resistant, pesticide resistant, and faster growing wheat than we have today, it has to be hybridized," this is where the genetic engineering comes into play. The result is an estimated **5%** or so of the original wheat proteins are **NEW**. Guess what this means to the body? It does not recognize it and as a result reacts with systemic inflammation. Remember the inflammatory markers I just spoke of, such as homocysteine? But first the immune system will also create anti-bodies to attack these unrecognizable proteins. In a celiac patient, who may even have silent Celiac's I spoke of earlier for instance, the anti-bodies also attack the tTG, the same enzyme that broke down the gluten to gliadin and glutenin to begin with. The job of this enzyme is also to bind or hold together the cell junctions in your intestines so nothing can get through; it also increases the surface area of the intestines with microvilli, hairy finger like projections, so nutrients can be absorbed. If this enzyme designed to protect the intestines gets attacked, your microvilli will shrink and deteriorate so that your body cannot absorb nutrients. This is what occurs in Celiac's. This leads to the microvilli becoming leaky. **The gluten can also cause the cells lining your intestine to secrete a protein called zonulin which breaks down the tight borders binding your intestines together**. Alas, we now have *Leaky Gut Syndrome*. The leaky gut will then let undigested foods, toxins, and antibodies move throughout your body by way of the blood stream. Now your body will start attacking them as a foreign invader, and the autoimmune reaction is born. As Dr. Myers puts it, "This can manifest itself in digestive symptoms including bloating, constipation, diarrhea, and weight loss." Patients can also have malabsorption of fats including fatty acids and vitamin D and malnutrition issues, such as iron deficiency anemia. This sounds a lot like the thyroid issues I previously discussed, doesn't it? This is why gluten free is especially important to maintain thyroid health. Dr. Myers stresses that those with Celiac's autoimmune disease are at risk of getting another autoimmune disease for this reason. She recommends getting "screened for autoimmunity if you are gluten intolerant."

In other words, the leaky gut allowing the undigested proteins to go through your bloodstream and travel to different areas of your body can lead to painful symptoms that you are ascribing to other causes. For example, the gluten can travel to your joints causing joint paints that you may mistake for just arthritis. Many people experience symptoms and misdiagnose their causes, unaware that the true source is **gluten**. I find that almost everybody I have tested is autoimmune so my advice is STAY AWAY FROM GLUTEN.

Most of the criticism of a gluten free diet is a lack of fiber resulting. Adding things like chia seeds, more water intake in between meals, and eating or drinking dark green leafy vegetables, however, will more than make up for the loss of fiber in a gluten free diet and is much healthier. If you are currently cooking with wheat or white flour, however, switch to almond, coconut, garbanzo bean, or brown rice flour. Keep in mind that there are still antibodies for up to six months after you stop eating gluten, but for many of you a trial period of at least one, and more likely three months, will be sufficient to notice the life changing benefits. If you re-introduce gluten into diet, you will notice how much better you felt without it. Re-read the dangers of gluten and then give the gluten free diet a try. August 1, 2013, marked the finalization of the FDA's Gluten Free Labeling Regulation assuring all consumers that all products labeled gluten-free in the United States must follow standardized governmental guidelines. Another tiny step forward……

My wife found a great free iPhone app called, "shop well." You can set the app based on general health preferences such as diabetes, weight management, athletic training and so on. In addition, you can set the app to filter out foods containing one of or a combination of unwanted categories, like gluten, dairy, soy, etc. After scanning a food, your phone will then respond with poor, good, or excellent choice based on your chosen categories. Keep in mind; this is only for foods which are in the program. There are so many brands on the market that some barcodes will show "not recognized" after you scan them. I found this app excellent when you are not sure about the ingredients of certain foods. After you have been shopping this way for a while, you will probably not need this app. There is also a website, www.whatcontainsgluten.com, which can provide more information on good shopping choices. Recently, I stumbled across another site showing a table that determines the extent of how "gluten free" certain brands of food are, in other words how many parts per million (ppm) of gluten they contain. Many of the so called "gluten free" foods are not truly totally free of gluten but just have traces which will not bother many with gluten sensitivity, but will not be advisable for celiac patients. We also have to remember "silent Celiac's" here. The link for this info is: http://celiacdisease.about.com/od/PreventingCrossContamination/a/Gluten-Free-PPM-table.htm.

You must try to avoid all of the GMO foods you can. Our cells do not recognize genetically modified foods and are more prone, therefore, to attack them as invaders causing an unfolding cascade of auto immune events. **A good way to "try" and avoid GMO foods is to buy only 100% organic products which are supposedly not allowed to contain any GMOS**. These products are *supposed* to not be allowed to contain GMOs. However, a "made with organic ingredients" label only require 70% of the ingredients to be organic and may not be GMO free, another example of manufacturer's attempts to evade or camouflage the real ingredients. Organic certification, however, is a USDA certification program standard; unfortunately its meaning is becoming continually more ambiguous, and its standards less stringent due to large food corporations wanting in on the extremely lucrative "organic" market.

I suppose 70% organic is better than 0% organic. Trying to buy GMO free products is the right thing to do even if you are duped by deceptive marketing. Otherwise, you would be just turning a blind eye and hoping for the best. The latter choice will not lead to organic and non-GMO foods getting into your diet. I know buying organic products is more costly, but you cannot put a price on your long term health. Besides, if you reduce the amount of the junk in your diet you will have more money to buy good nutritious foods that your body really needs. Also look for "non GMO" labels and avoid products made with crops that are GMO. Usually this is from the "Big Four:" corn, soybeans, canola, and cottonseed-used in processed foods. For example, some of the most common ingredients in corn, one of the Big Four in processed foods are: corn flour, corn meal, corn oil, corn starch, corn syrup, sweeteners such as fructose, dextrose, and glucose, and modified food starch. The "buffer zone" for non-GMO corn is usually meaningless today, however, because corn can cross-pollinate for miles; thus some GMO corn DNA is found in organic certified corn. The sad truth is that GMO corn makes up to 90% of the US corn crop. Considering soy, products are: soy flour, soy lecithin, soy protein, soy isolate, soy isoflavone, vegetable oil and vegetable protein. Go back to the earlier section where I talked about soy and you will see why you should avoid it. Look out for canola or rapeseed oil and cottonseed they are garbage oils.

Meat, fish, and fowl that are GMO are NOT YET approved in this country for human consumption. Remember "Frankenfish" and how GMO companies are trying to get it in the market as soon as possible. Yet many non-organic foods are produced from animals raised on GMO foods like grains. Buy grass fed beef and wild caught fish to avoid farmed fish fed on a GMO diet. There are alternative meat products which are processed and may include GMO ingredients. Carefully read label ingredients and look for the Big Four at risk ingredients, most notably, soy.

Baby formulas are mostly made out of soy and milk. That milk is usually from cows injected with rbGH, aka growth hormone. A lot of the brands also contain GMO-derived corn syrup, corn syrup solids, or soy lecithin. Try a rice-based formula if not breast-feeding and again look for the Big Four ingredients.

Dairy products may also be filled with growth hormone from injected cows to boost milk production. Please reject the "lack of calcium" argument from dairy farmers promoting their product; investigation will find that the health benefit claims are suspect. If you insist on drinking cow's milk, organic dairy products are growth hormone free and do not use GMO grains as feed so buy them. Be aware that products with labels indicating the cows were growth hormone free may still be from cows that were fed GMO feed. Most alternative "dairy free" products are made from soybeans, one of the Big Four, and may also contain GMO materials.

Only use glass baby bottles and not plastic due to the Bisphenol A leaching out of these bottles labeled with the recycling codes 3 or 7. Pregnant women should DEFINATELY avoid these plastics because the unborn child is more susceptible than adults to the effects of BPH. I must note that all pregnant women should buy a book titled, "How to Raise a Healthy Child in Spite of your Doctor," by Robert Mendelsohn

MD. Although it is not sold in stores anymore, it is available online and will save you many trips to the doctor's office.

Breakfast cereals and bars are most likely to contain GMO ingredients such as corn and soy and, in my opinion, are junk. The *"Organic Food Bar"* the brand PRL sells is an exception; if you are eating cold cereal for breakfast, you are not eating as healthy as you should. These are too processed and turn to sugar immediately. Remember my breakfast choice on weekdays? Non GMO, organic, gluten free oatmeal; give it a try.

Baked goods usually contain corn syrup, which is GMO and also trans-fatty acids to keep them on the shelf longer. Frozen foods can be highly processed. Again, look out for the Big Four GMO ingredients. This is also true for soups, sauces, and canned foods. The latter can also be loaded with large amounts of table salt rather than the desired nutritious pink sea salt.

Condiments, oils, salad dressings, and spreads probably contain GMO ingredients. Try to find an organic salad dressing that is non GMO, gluten free, with no added sugar or soy, and free of junk oils. For oils, choose pure extra virgin olive oil, coconut oil, sesame oil, and almond oil. There are great recipes online to make your own salad dressing. For example, you can use a combination of virgin olive oil, Bragg's brand raw apple cider vinegar, PRL's *pink salt*, and black pepper. If you buy jelly, get it made with pure cane sugar and not corn syrup. Just do not eat too much as the glycemic index is high.

When you buy sugar, remember ANYTHING NOT LISTED AS 100% CANE SUGAR may be derived from other sources and definitely will adversely affect your blood sugar levels. Make sure you look for organic and non-GMO sweeteners, candy and chocolate products made with 100% cane sugar, evaporated cane juice or organic sugar to avoid GMO beet sugar, which recently flooded the sugar market.

Remember, that the herb Stevia is the best choice for a sugar substitute because it does not spike your blood sugar. Many people do not like the taste of Stevia, however, so they should use organic cane sugar in small amounts at one sitting. All other substitute sugars, including Aspartame, (NutraSweet) and Equal, found in over 6,000 products like soft drinks, gum, candy, desserts, and many yogurts, are toxic chemicals that must be avoided.

Speaking of gum and mints, there was an excellent article my wife read to me this morning, on www.naturalnews.com, explaining that just strolling down the checkout isle at the grocery store can be hazardous to your health if you buy sugar free gum, mints, and candy on display there thinking this is a wise choice. The fact is you either have a choice of getting pesticide infested corn syrup with the sweetened kind or the "nervous-wreck" sugar free kind containing aspartame. I note this only because I see people who chew a lot of gum and eat these mints all day long, not thinking of their chemical dangers. Watch the gluten in a lot of gum brands; remember when any food are listed as "gluten free" it only needs to mean less than 20 parts per million so it is not really gluten free.

Sodas and fruit juices, lacking fiber necessary to slow down their digestion, also contain high amounts of the GMO based high fructose corn syrup. When you drink orange or apple juice it is the equivalent of eating a bunch of oranges or apples at one time without the healthy fiber they contain. Remember it can sit for up to a year in tanks before it reaches the supermarket. Google it for yourself and you will be amazed. The "freshly squeezed" taste claims on the orange juice commercials are very misleading; it is not fresh oranges used by any stretch of the imagination. To keep the juice from spoiling producers remove the oxygen and with it goes the natural flavor of the oranges. Casey Chan, at Gizmodo Company, explains that drink companies hire flavor and fragrance companies, the same ones that make perfume for Dior, to create the flavor pack that makes the oxygen deprived liquid taste like juice again. Other juice and soda companies who use the flavor packs are: Tropicana (owned by PepsiCo), Minute Maid (Coca Cola), Simply Orange (also Coca Cola), and independently owned Florida's Natural. Minute Maid is said to have a candy-like orange flavor because producers choose a Coca Cola flavor pack for it. How is that for deception? Remember the commercial where the lady at the supermarket reaches into the freezer and on the other side someone is handing her freshly squeezed orange juice from oranges just picked. Keep these deceptive ad practices in mind when watching all of those ridiculous cereal commercials and their false health claims as well.

Avoid drinking all of these sugary caffeine laden energy drinks, such as sodas and lattes. Because Starbucks sells mainly these non-nutritious drinks, they should not be a thriving business. Furthermore, all of these caffeine drinks dehydrate you and cause more inflammation. Many in this country are continually partially dehydrated as a result of too much caffeine and lack of water consumption. Remember each 8 ounces of coffee demands 32 ounces of water to process it. Begin drinking a lot of water, but not from the tap (remember the fluoride) or vitamin enhanced water, that contains 32 grams of sugar the arch enemy of good health.

With good spring or well water drink half your bodyweight in ounces. It deserves repeating; you need to be able to flush out the daily toxins that we unknowingly and knowingly ingest. The water will also help you achieve your ideal weight. Try to drink out of a glass container ideally and if plastic, make sure it is BPH free certified.

After all of the research on dieting and what works, it all comes down to this: calories in versus calories out. If you are not burning the calories you eat you will gain weight; burn more calories than you ingest and you will lose weight. Again remember, most packaged "diets" are based on a limited number of calories and for convenience sake. You eat the "non-nutritive pseudo food" that is shipped to you and lose the weight. However, this is not a lifestyle change. You are not taught how to use and prepare foods properly after the pre-packaged weight loss phase is over. And many people do not stay with "fad diets" for very long and will regain the weight. A serious diet counts calories, allows few starches and very minimal amounts of sugars. Weight will usually fly off people when they give up the grains and starches such as breads, pastas, potatoes and white rice - really any type of flour. This is the diet I recommend. Look at the "PALEO" diet with some modifications but not necessarily as extreme. I do eat brown rice and potatoes, sweet potatoes and occasionally foods breaded with a gluten free breading, but I stay away from any added sugars. Try to be strict on weekdays and relax more on the weekends. I constantly hear patients say they lost twenty or even thirty pounds by simply NOT EATING AS MUCH AS THEY WERE. They add, "I simply ate about one half of the usual portions I was eating." If you go to the restaurant, take half of it home for the next day. All of the diets available will usually result in temporary weight loss; however, only a true LIFESTYLE change with SENSIBLE eating will keep you at your ideal weight and health. Some great recipes are available at www.paleOMG.com.

In my Holistic practice, we have a workable weight loss Patients fill out a comprehensive questionnaire on the initial visit which also evaluates their health concerns. After five weeks on the program, they will fill it out again to assess progress; at this point a patient can do another weight loss phase to lose more weight if needed. On the other hand, if they have lost all the weight they need to; we now address some of their other health concerns. We find that during the re-assessment, however, many of the original health concerns have disappeared or improved. They could be food sensitivities and/or detoxification ability, for example, which contributed to their previous overweightness in the first place. Finally, when all of the health issues have been addressed and their metabolism has been re-balanced to burn calories more efficiently, patients go on a stabilization phase so that their hypothalamus (part of the brain) will re-set to their new weight. This will ensure no weight gain after the re-introduction of some of the foods avoided during the weight loss phase; if re-introducing foods after the weight loss without stabilizing or addressing other health concerns, the yo-yo diet problem results.

Having said all of that, I do occasionally get a patient who has done the 1200-calorie diet on his own without any supplements and has not lost any weight. If you diet on your own, my advice is to get your metabolism typed. Read the Wolcott and Fahey book I discussed earlier titled "The Metabolic Typing Diet." According to Fahey, some of you will do better with protein and fats and some with carbohydrates; others will be lucky enough to do the best with a combination of all three. If someone has more of a carbohydrate metabolic type and goes on a 1200-calorie minimal carbohydrate diet, how do you think he is going to feel? Unfortunately, one size diet does not fit all.

As I stated earlier, there is a huge problem with chronic low stomach acid in this country. Again, we look at the starches and sugars which REDUCE its production needed to digests protein foods. So when you combine sugars and starches with proteins and you have a low stomach acid problem, the undigested food sits in the gastrointestinal tract and putrefies leading to a lot of digestion complaints including reflux and the formation of AGE's leading to neurodegeneration. When it comes to achieving or maintaining a healthy weight do what my wife tells me when I am trying to be a handy man around the house: "Work smarter not harder." The weight loss system in place at my office exemplifies this last statement. We have a set protocol with proven results. If you have a history of weight problems, research has shown it is too hard to stay on track by doing it yourself. You will learn how to keep weight off, what to do if the pounds creep up, and how to eat healthy. Not to mention YOU HAVE TO BE ACCOUNTABLE TO SOMEONE - *ME!* I will conclude the weight loss topic with this last statement. THERE IS NO MAJIC TO WEIGHT LOSS, JUST HARD WORK AND DEDICATION. Remember, I am not referring to those unfortunate few with leptin resistance who cannot lose weight no matter what they do. And remember, also body fat loves toxins. When you begin to lose the weight you may feel worse as the toxins leave your body. Do not get discouraged; it will pass.

Sometimes it is not just about what to eat, breathe in, or rub into your skin to make you healthier, but WHAT ENVIORMENTAL substances YOU SHOULD AVOID. For instance, many of you will be exposed to harsh chemicals like cigarette smoke or some type of chemical fumes at work. If you cannot get away from it, you must take some free radical supplements for systemic inflammation. Look at the section of this book where I talked about the need for maintenance or grocery list of supplements that we should take daily.

I get a chuckle out of those people who smoke, for instance, and then take vitamin C reasoning that it negates all of the adverse effects of the smoke. Remember smoking KILLS 85% of its users in the end. Try to quit; if you have tried before, try harder. Because it takes motivation find something that you really want and give it to yourself when you reach your smoke-free goals. You need the support of your friends and family to do this. Smokers, along with alcoholics and the morbidly obese all have addictive personalities and this cannot be neglected. You will probably trade in one vice for another when you quit smoking, such as eating too much. Be addicted to something beneficial, such as fitness for example or another activity you always wanted to pursue.

We should all have some reserve against the constant bombardment of free radicals we are up against with our food system and environment. Remember, times of stress will deplete your vitamins and minerals while exploiting any bodily weakness. I am willing to test anyone with QRA to see exactly what their bodies need. Even if you test strong for a certain supplement, having a reserve of nutrients for all of the daily stressors is beneficial.

Let's talk about the effects of stress on the body with a simple analogy. Think of a bucket of water. When the bucket is too full the water overflows. Consider the water as stress, and when the water spills over the side of the bucket, we have the symptoms of high stress caused by all stressors, physical, mental, chemical. GMO foods, gluten and soy for example, are three major stressors we can eliminate from our diet with a little patience.

The personal hygiene products we rub into our skin on a daily basis and the house cleaners we inhale are chemical stressors we can easily eliminate. Therefore, if we can eliminate enough of these stressors, the water (stress) level will be low and any weakness that your body has to stress will not be exploited. Try switching your toothpaste, deodorant, shampoo, facial cleanser, facial cream, and other personal hygiene products to those without the toxic chemicals. Cleaning supplies also have many toxic chemicals and are often estrogenic; see if you can find substitutes. There is a "Mrs. Meyer's" hardworking household cleaner's brand you can investigate. Many products can be found on the Internet; you can even find recipes for making your own cleaners such as dishwashing and laundry detergent. Becky recently made her own laundry detergent which works well and is free of the harmful chemicals and strong fragrances. It consists of washing soda, borax and castile soap with essential oils and makes 5 gallons at a time. Look for natural ingredient cleaners. Many natural household cleaners use lemons and oranges as they are a great astringent.

Start to replace your plastic food storage containers with glass mason jars. Plastic containers can leach chemicals into the food.

Don't wait until after you are diagnosed with a severe disease to switch to safer products. Substituting with less toxic chemicals is only common sense. Even though you think you are doing well, most of the products we use in this country are extremely toxic. Having an industrialized nation comes at a cost. Financial gain is first priority, our health second.

Let me stop here and interject that I know a lot of you reading this may be saying to yourself, "I am not worried about the chemicals in cleaning products. That is just too intense or obsessive." That is fine. I am not that strict on cleaning products either because I know that there are so many other harmful substances to avoid. However, the toxins in cleaning products are estrogenic, mimicking the harmful effects of estrogen dominance. This is NOT good. The majority of cleaning product users are women and if you are suffering from PMS, heavy bleeding, fibroids, you may want to change to more natural cleaning products. You can also cut out something else that is unhealthy or add a healthy one. Remember, it is a give and take with becoming healthier. **You need to reduce the toxic load your body is exposed to on a daily basis.** For instance, do not be someone whose diet consists of nothing but junk food i.e. soda, donuts, pop tarts, and also worries if your corn is GMO? The soda, donuts, and pop tarts will probably kill you faster than the GMO corn. Do the research and make logical choices here; just be sure you are coming out ahead on the healthy side. Hopefully, throughout this book I have given you a lot of examples how to accomplish this.

I mentioned an article earlier on the dangers of mercury fillings and having two different metals in your mouth, such as a crown, bridge, or mercury fillings forming a galvanic current which leeches mercury from your mouth at a much faster rate than normal into your tissues.

Ideally, we should have no metal in our mouths, but if that cannot be accomplished we should only have one kind. I plan to have my mercury fillings removed and replaced with amalgam fillings. For this you need to find a holistic dentist.

Try to get a half an hour of sun per day when the weather permits; it is good for you. If you are in a bathing suit for about thirty minutes your body will make its VIT D for the day. For those out in the sun a lot longer, use a natural sunblock. Rubbing those chemical laden sunscreens in your skin and your children's skin is not good. Look up the ingredients on the Internet, and you will be surprised what you are rubbing into your body. When the cold months come, you can still get your body to make VIT D using a Mercola tanning bed. I know most people think tanning beds are not good and cause skin cancer but you will be pleasantly surprised at what Dr. Mercola says about tanning beds in one of his articles.

Dr. Mercola says it is "ultraviolet light that causes your skin to convert cholesterol into vitamin D. It is possible to get UVB, good rays, from a tanning bed, but the EMFs produced by magnetic ballasts used by the vast majority of tanning beds are of major concern. You must make sure you're using a tanning bed that employs newer electronic ballasts, which virtually eliminate this risk and are safe. They also use about 30 percent less electricity and produce more light, so they are far more economical to run." On the subject of ultraviolet rays causing Melanoma, the conventional wisdom has been that sun's exposure is the culprit. Yet research published by the British Journal of Dermatology reveals that the sun is likely "nothing more than a scapegoat in the development of Melanoma." This is like the way cholesterol is blamed for all of the heart attacks and strokes. You see there is something called diagnostic drift by which researchers believe that there has been a steady rise in the misdiagnosis of non-cancerous lesions erroneously classified as Stage 1 Melanoma.

He continues to state that "exposure to sunlight, particularly UVB, is actually *protective* against melanoma—or rather, the vitamin D your body produces in response to UVB radiation is protective." Go to Dr. Mercola's website and see for yourself. You can also just take 6 drops of *Serum d3* from PRL to get your daily dose of Vit D.

Speaking of misdiagnosis, I was floored when looking on the Johnson forum recently. I discovered a post by Dr. Linda Ehlers. She discussed a report commissioned by the U.S. National Cancer Institute (NCI) that stated, "**A significant number of people who have undergone treatment for cancer over the past several decades may not have ever actually had the disease.** Published online in the Journal of the American Medical Association (JAMA), this government study identifies both over diagnosis and misdiagnosis of cancer as two major causes of the growing cancer epidemic..." Wow.

Remember how I grounded my house and office for EMF protection and used the Q-disc. I am sure everybody has heard that scientists first said that the brain is not affected by EMF's. More recently, they flip-flopped and said it is probably not a good idea to hold a cell phone up to your ear for any length of time, nor is it is a good idea to live within a certain radius from a cell phone tower. An article on the Johnson forum posted by Dr. Walter Crooks, explained that there were 7,000 cancer deaths linked to cell phone towers. The research was done in Brazil. Moreover, Dr. Oz advised woman on his television show, not to put their cell phones in their shirt because they could increase their chances for breast cancer. This is bad news. If you do not have a hands free phone device or are on the cell phone a lot, get a Q disc that sticks to the back of your phone and will stop the EMF's from going into your brain. It is available from PRL for $80. Ground your house protecting your family from EMFs both cheaply and easily with a bag of *Dragonite;* a twenty pound bag is $30.00.

I did not get a flu shot. After researching this highly controversial topic, I did not feel that any so called benefit was worth the risk. Concerning vaccinations get the "A Shot in the Dark" book I alluded to earlier and then make up your own mind. And when the kids are teenagers you may have to decide on the Gardasil vaccine.

Make sure you are getting enough sleep. Many people do not get into deep REM (rapid eye movement) uninterrupted sleep needed for whole body healing. Just resting and lying around is great for the body but it does not help the mind to function properly the next day. Most people know how many hours of sleep they need; try to get that amount. If you have trouble sleeping or staying asleep you probably have stomach and gallbladder issues. Furthermore, if you wake up tired, your adrenal glands need support. In other words, if you balance your metabolism you will sleep much better.

In view of everything I have said up unto this point, would you not agree it is probably better to try a conservative approach to preventative health **first** versus an invasive drug/surgery approach? This advice is for a person who does not know the cause of their health concern and is simply covering it up with symptomatic medications hoping for the best. I hope I have made the case thus far that this is probably not a good idea if you want to achieve and maintain ideal health.

Thus, I strongly recommend that people investigate chiropractic or naturopathic medicine. You can go to the medical specialist first to get checked out. Get all of the expensive, and often unnecessary, diagnostic tests to satisfy any worry you have about something seriously wrong.

 Before you do any invasive medical treatment, however, think about first giving someone in the natural field a chance. Some chiropractors are also well versed in nutrition and others are not. You can explore their website or call and ask questions. In my office, as I previously discussed, we also offer many other therapies besides chiropractic. For example, I see many patients for laser, QRA, and functional medicine, and weight loss.

Keep in mind a chiropractors goal is to return you to better health. Again, consider visiting one so you can achieve your health goals together instead of just taking a symptom-suppressing pill and thinking everything is just fine, as the drug industry wants you to believe. Remember, however, disease is not due to a drug deficiency and good health is not achieved from taking prescription drugs. Now I am not taking about a drug someone depends on daily or they would die such as insulin for Type1 diabetes, or an epi-pen for anaphylactic shock, or many other serious life threatening illnesses, I am talking about the preventable disease drug merry go round. Another quote from Dr. Mercola's article on the documentary, "Pill Poppers:" "The difference between a drug and poison is the dose."

An important point to remember: You *can* feel immediate changes with supplements but you will *almost always* feel immediate changes from taking prescription or over the counter medication that only block pain receptors in your brain. The goal of natural, drug-free nutritional supplements, on the other hand, is to balance out your body systems so it can take care of itself on its own. They do not work simply by suppressing pain and symptoms like medications do and take longer to be effective. If you just want to take a pill and forget about it or if you only want to lead a very sedentary lifestyle eating mostly junk food, let's just say you should go the medical route and pop the pills. I trying to be reasonable here; the drug free low sugary simple carbohydrate lifestyle is not for everybody. Although everybody wants the benefits of living a healthy lifestyle; sadly only a few will take the necessary actions to achieve them.

Of course there are instances when drugs and hospitals are necessary. First I want to briefly mention back and neck pain because, as I said earlier, that is what most people will go to a chiropractor for. I am very experienced and knowledgeable at treating lower back and neck pain, especially with disc cases. I ask patients to give me three visits per week for two weeks or six visits. If they are not showing any significant improvement then I send them medical doctor for drugs, physical therapy etc. For example, my wife just recently aggravated her lower back. I tried everything; laser, decompression, flexion distraction, adjustments, and ice, multiple times per day to try and calm down the inflammation around the nerve. But the treatments were not enough to get ahead of the inflammation. Therefore, I called an orthopedic surgeon's office and got her prednisone (a corticosteroid anti-inflammatory) which she took for a week and got about 95% better. Sometimes the drugs are the only thing that will work to get the patient over the hump but I always try the conservative approach first because usually it works without the risk of side effects. The same goes for organic type symptoms. When someone presents with both very severe and ambiguous symptoms that just do not add up and are not mechanical, or affected by movement, it is time to send that person to the emergency room. This is especially true with the warning signs of a stroke, heart attack, gall bladder attack, kidney stone or attack. **It is always better to be safe than sorry**.

Thus, for those of you looking for answers to be healthier, don't succumb to the drug industry's hype and simply take numerous potential harmful medications each morning. As I hope I explained throughout this book, **most chronic diseases are largely preventable with SIMPLE LIFESTYLE CHANGES**. You can stay well naturally, without the use of drugs and frequent conventional medical/disease care. This is, in fact, the most successful strategy you can use to gain longevity. For example, instead of an aspirin a day as a preventative measure for "heart health," look into taking turmeric. There is a lot of new information on the power of turmeric; it can replace 15 drugs from anti-inflammatories to aspirin. If you can substitute a drug for something natural and in most cases equally or more effective, then doesn't it make sense to do so? Of course, you must always read the contraindications of your prescription drugs with any nutritional supplements you plan to take. If a natural substance does what the drug is supposed to do without the side effects - why not? Do not expect to get this tip from your family doctor; you have to be proactive and research this on your own.

If you are recently diagnosed with a debilitating illness or even cancer **you need to take action right now. You don't take your car in for an oil change after you blow the engine do you?** You need to totally change your lifestyle. Remember the adage, doing the same thing over and over and expecting different results is insanity? Well, it was those SAME things that you have always done or neglected to that allowed your body to succumb to the disease or cancer in the first place. To heal, you need to TOTALLY CHANGE YOUR DIETARY HABITS AND LIFESTYLE. THIS SHOULD BE COMMON SENSE but in this country we are too brainwashed by Big Pharma and the medical community to use logic. Unfortunately, there are those few cases where a cancer or illness is developed due to unforeseeable factors such as genetics such as a child born with a terminal defect. I am not referring to these poor souls; they need medical treatment.

I know that many reading this may think it is a lot of work to try to be healthier. **You are right. It does take a lot of work.** It is easy to fall into the routine of TV dinners, all processed foods, sugary drinks, lattes, soda, a lot of prescription and over the counter drugs, no exercise, and minimal water consumption. And if you around, there is always rationalization for any unhealthy behavior you are engaged in. Remember, I said it a million times, "PEOPLE TAKE THE PATH OF

LEAST RESISTANCE." Try to use some of the energy you expend on a daily basis developing unhealthy habits to actually do something good for yourself. You will feel better once you clean up your diet. You need to also exercise five times per week, if possible. Go for a walk over your lunch break and work up to an hour of walking per day if you do nothing else. While watching TV, you can use a portable pedal device-ergometer for twenty to thirty minutes, while watching television or while sitting on a chair to exercise your legs or arms. There are exercise bands that also allow you to watch television while you use them; you will not even feel like you are exercising. Gold's gym even has a movie theater room with cardio machines instead of chairs to keep your mind distracted while you exercise. You will have more energy and will want to be more active when you begin to exercise.

I must mention something here that I think will make a huge difference in your life and could save you a lot of future problems with your back, neck, and extremities. I am talking about trying to become more ambidextrous, as I mentioned earlier, using both hands interchangeably. Remember, due to all of the twisting in daily activities, right-handers wear out the left annulus or ligament part of the disk between your vertebras conversely left-handed people wear out the right annulus. When shoveling snow for example, rest your elbow on your knee so you are not putting too much strain on your back and then switch hands after a few minutes. The same is true for your neck and turning your head. If you are a forklift operator and turn your head 1,000 times to the left, you need to also turn your head to the other direction or to the right that same day. You could do some right rotation exercises with isometrics later that evening. Twisting and turning may not affect the disk as much in the neck as in the lower back but it will affect the muscles, ligaments, and tendons by shortening them and causing imbalance. There are the repetitive activities that people do with their hands. From a factory worker to a secretary, using only the dominant hand will make you more prone to not only sprain/strains of the muscles, tendons, ligaments, but it could lead to something more serious.

Now I am going to think outside the box on this one. Being ambidextrous can also help with restoring balance to both sides of the brain when one side is showing a decreased frequency of firing. In other words, if your right front brain is decreased and you are right handed, you could be causing more of an imbalance when doing certain activities. So you need to really make a conscious effort to do activities using either hand interchangeably.

Try to also lift objects by maintain correct posture. The three cardinal rules for safe lifting are: Keep the load close, bend your knees, and keep your nose between your toes to avoid twisting. Remember, when you hold something out in front of you, your lower back is the anchor and takes all of the stress. You may have seen an older man walk with the forward head posture. Usually they also have chronic lower back pain. I must also mention activities like ironing and vacuuming can also result in lower back pain. Women could actually wash dishes and iron while putting one foot on a small step stool taking pressure off the lower back. When vacuuming, remember not to take big strokes or strides; I remember a woman who did this and ended up in the ambulance with a ruptured disk. Vacuuming is very provocative for lower back pain. If after any activity, you begin to feel sore or are starting to stiffen up, you need to apply ice to the affected area. There is continual disagreement over the use of ice and heat for pain. While it is true that heat increases brain firing and ice decreases it, I am mostly referring to recent trauma or chronic musculoskeletal pain patients who experience shooting pain down the arm or leg, for example; they need ice. For my chronic disease patients such as those suffering with dizziness, or fibromyalgia, I will use heat. I will say for the musculoskeletal pain cases, ice has definitely given me **FAR** superior results over heat the past twenty-five years.

When you are stuck in the daily grind of following the herd, so to speak, you develop a brain fog that makes it hard to act like you used to when you were younger and healthier, before all of the junk in the food and environment wore you down. Even though now the country is creating a bunch of zombie-like robots with the S.A.D., you have to rise above it; do not pity yourself. My dad taught me that while there is always someone better off than you out there, there is also someone worse off than you. Look at my buddy John for example. He suffered a debilitating stroke 15 years or so ago and told me that he cried himself to sleep every night for a year not knowing if he would ever walk again, let alone exercise. BUT HE PERSEVERED; he could have given up and just sat there saying "poor me" but he did not. And as a result he has both my respect and admiration. Just think of his story when you are not motivated enough to start exercising.

My wife Becky and I were out at a restaurant with John and his wife Tori last year, and we were amazed at how many people would came up to John and wanted to hug him and talk to him. A man who used to workout at Gold's when John and Tori owned it, told John how he

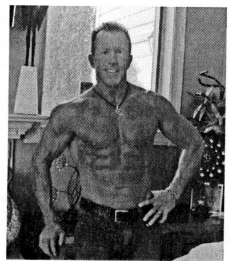

was inspired by him. I remember John telling me one time how his wife Tori was a little disgusted when going over the membership drop off rate. It appears that most gym members would only last for a few months and then quit. She turned to him and said, "Look at you - you even had a stroke and you still show up daily." Now John just recently had to undergo

Figure 2: John 14 years after a stroke. How is that for 57 years old?

right hip replacement surgery. I knew he would be training as soon as possible because this is just another bump in the road for him to step over. Only six weeks after surgery he was back in the gym. I did give him an intense two weeks dose of *Nucleoimmune* and *Aloe Mannin-Fx* supplements to take immediately after surgery. He went for his checkup today and the doctor said in only nine weeks, since the surgery, he is at the level most patients are at after six months post-surgery! I like to relate this philosophy of life to a scene in the movie *Predator* where Jessie Ventura's character was shot. Someone said, "You're bleeding." Jessie's character replied, "I ain't got time to bleed." That sums it up, people. You have to have discipline and drive to just get it done. Just hoping and dreaming are fine for fairy tales, but they will not change your life. **Change requires action.**

We all have to take responsibility for our own health. It is not the government or insurance company's responsibility, but yours and mine. You have to EDUCATE YOURSELF. Do not be fooled into thinking that the government would not let anything happen to you, that all of these harmful chemicals I have talked about could not be that bad because the government would not allow anyone to harm us. Well just look at the drug Vioxx. The FDA is known for their ineffective screenings and blatant conflict of interest. They failed to take Vioxx off the market until it killed 55,000 people. Many of the FDA workers are former drug company and food industry executives.

Well there you have it. This is a lot of information to process. I thoroughly enjoyed putting this down on paper; it allowed me to purge over twenty years of frustration in dealing with the shortsightedness of the medical mindset. If you got ANYTHING at all out of this book, then it was worth it to me. I hope you are not overwhelmed on how to start becoming healthier. Just re-read some sections and try to change your life for the better by implementing one "healthier" thing at a time.

Look, we all heard of those who smoke, drink, and eat junk and still live to be 90 years old. Just like we all knew of those who lived what seemed to be a stellar lifestyle, only to die young. So what does it all mean? Nobody knows. There is no crystal ball to look into. Research today, however, is leaning more towards nurture or the fact that genes can be changed by environment and lifestyle. Thus, I tried to provide you with as much information as I can about what is healthy and what is not healthy or harmful to your body. But we only live once and should have fun in life. The hard part then is to balance the things that are good for you versus those that are not so good. You have to make up your own mind on what foods and chemicals you want in your bodies and how far you want to go with a healthier lifestyle. But regardless of what you decide, at least you now know many of the seemingly innocent things that are indeed harming you. I hope you also now know many of the changes that will help you, or should I say at least you now know there are many things which may require further investigation. From this time forward, please do not use the excuse that you do not know what to do to become healthier.

I am going to wrap it up now. I could go on and on with this. I am sure my 12th grade English teacher would say, "Watch the lack of cohesion." It is indeed how he signed my yearbook.

I hope I painted a picture of how BIG MONEY really decides health care policy and what we, the public, are exposed to. You have to weed through all of the misleading advertising and shadily sponsored research. Really folks, I do not want to come off like a conspiring crazy person. I am not implying that the government and drug companies are blatantly saying, "The heck with the health of the American public." It is just that food and drug companies are funding studies exaggerating any benefit while turning a blind eye towards the detrimental effects of their products by using washout periods. I am just looking for the truth about health in a world where you have to somehow look beyond greed and deceit to find it. Much of the information I used in this book is from doctors throughout the country on the Johnson forum. These doctors are extremely bright and generously share their findings and research with all of us on the board. This enabled me to offer, you the public, the latest cutting edge information. I want to take the opportunity to thank all of these doctors again. Go to www.lifechangingcare.com to locate a Johnson Group doctor near you. There is a lot of information on the site along with many satisfied patient testimonials.

I also want to add that I do not receive any benefit or kickbacks from any of the products, companies, or doctors I mentioned in this book. I just want to give you the best information I can so that you can make the most informed decision. I care more about you reaching your ideal health than I do about the bottom line.

Finally, get on the internet and research some of this information; do not just take my word for it. Here is a statement I remember reading from an unknown author which really sums it all up. "We spend our health in search of wealth, we toll, we sweat, we slave - then we spend our wealth in search of health but all we get is the grave." Again, do not wait too long to make a change for the better. No regrets. And when it comes to your health I hope you take a *Common "Sensible" Approach*!